<u>THIS</u> IS INSANITY!

This
Is
Insanity!

No Dieting • No Exercising
No Counseling • No Results
Stay the way you look
and feel – forever

by Beth Donahue

THE SUMMIT GROUP • FORT WORTH, TEXAS

PUBLISHED BY THE SUMMIT GROUP
1227 WEST MAGNOLIA, SUITE 500
FORT WORTH, TEXAS 76104

99 98 97 96 95 94   5 4 3 2 1

Library of Congress Cataloging-in-Publication Data

Donahue, Beth, 1962-
This is insanity!: no dieting, no exercising, no counseling, no results,
stay the way you look and feel forever / by Beth Donahue.
p. cm.
ISBN 1-56530-153-6: $9.95
1. Health—Humor. 2. Physical fitness—Humor. I. Title.
PN6231.H38D66 1994
818'.5402—dc20   94-32585
CIP

This Is Insanity! is a parody and a satire intended only for the fun, entertainment, and enjoyment of its readers. The materials in this book are not intended to provide medical, weight-loss, or any other health-related information, nor should they be relied upon to do so by the reader. References to specific products, people, and companies, or any other specific references, are included solely for the entertainment of the reader and are not to be taken as either endorsements or criticisms, nor should they be taken as describing actual facts or events.

Weight maintenance is a serious medical issue which should be dealt with only under the guidance of a physician or other professional trained in the areas of medical and mental health, health maintenance, or personal fitness.

Photography by Lloyd Poissenot

ACKNOWLEDGMENTS

I would like to thank the following people:

To my wonderful, funny, patient, dear, sweet, amazing parents, Don and Dee Donahue. I am so glad God chose you for me. I love you.

Elaine, Don, and Laura Lyn: thank you for always rooting for me and for being there.

Hayes Jackson, who spun straw into gold.

Brian Bradley, for being my best friend and the funniest person I know.

Dave Little, for making me laugh until I cry, and cry until I laugh, for making me laugh harder than anyone, and for being so amazingly kind at my worst moments. Thank you.

Dorothy Fischer, who brings me back from the brink of madness on a regular basis. My Anne Sullivan, I love you!

Brother Wease, Cindy, Tom, Charlie, Billy, and Stan the Man…thanks for fighting for me. You guys are the best. WCMF is the ONLY radio station!

The Fans in Rochester, New York. What can I say? Every one of you have touched my life in some way or another…thank you for your steadfast devotion, your gifts, letters, phone calls, faxes, and love. You guys are the BEST. Thank you.

Ross Rumberg, for spending an inhuman amount of time (and money!) trying to get me discovered, and for still liking me even after I looked at the files!

Melanie Ford, for all your legwork, and for trying harder than anyone I know. I love you, sweetie.

Randy Butler, for the first phone call.

Dr. Ed Tyska, for providing me with all the wonderful material! Thank you for all your help.

Jim Prochaska, Jennifer Hutton, and Lisa Carter of The Women's Total Fitness Center, for providing the first gym where it felt okay to be me.

Craig and Charlie Reed, The Proclaimers, for making the treadmill bearable because of your spectacular music, and for being astonishingly kind. You guys RULE! And special hugs to Tom Oliver.

Liz Bell and Brent Lockhart for talking me down...thanks.

Mike Towle, my editor, for being so patient with me!

Special thanks to: Gene McGuire, Leo Nino, Lori Hall, Joanna Pickens, Craig Lewis, Carol Baker, Gail Lacroix, Michael W. Smith, Mitch Kutash, and Gerard Fisher.

I would also like to thank God for not deserting me in my struggle to get closer to You.

This book is dedicated to the memory of my grandmother, Marion Brady, who finally is not in pain anymore.

CONTENTS

INTRODUCTION, 9

PART ONE • GETTING FAT

1 Tipping the Scales, 23
2 This Is All My Parents' Fault…Isn't It? 35

PART TWO • BEING FAT

3 You Know You're Fat When . . ., 43
4 Eating Wrong, 53
5 I Never Met a Diet I Liked, 67
6 101 Creative Recipes for Cardboard, 107
7 <u>Never</u> Consult a Physician, 115
8 <u>No One</u> Looks Good in a Thong, 129

PART THREE • DEALING WITH FAT

9 There's So Much of Me to Love, 159
10 Tricks of the Trade, 171
11 Climbing the Mountain—Yourself, 197
12 Questions and Answers, 207
13 Odds and (Rear) Ends, 217

AFTERWORD • 225

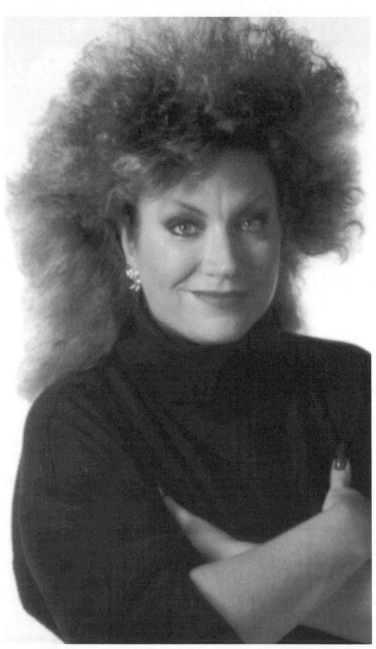

Me today…starving as usual.

INTRODUCTION

God created you in His own image.
Who knew there was so much of Him to go around?

I'm not angry, damn it!

I'm hungry!

Here I am, all 230 pounds of me, swaying back and forth in front of the refrigerator at 4:30 A.M., not even remotely hungry, but driven by some unseen force, determined to find something sweet to eat! I've looked under the bed, and all I found was an empty birthday cake box. Well, alright, I admit it—there were five of them. My bakery must think I'm insane; I told them I was a party planner so they wouldn't get suspicious when I order a birthday cake every week. The only problem is, I'm running out of names to put on the cakes. Believe it or not, there aren't that many Ishmaels and Ezekiels living in Dallas.

Wouldn't you know it, nothing in the fridge. Miss Smartypants decided to remove all the sweets from the house. But, it's amazing what you can come up with when you're a compulsive eater, isn't it? All of a sudden, I spy my old—and I do mean old—friend. There, on the bottom shelf behind the forty boxes of old

Jenny Haag food I never ate, is a can of chocolate syrup I bought right after the U.S. hockey team beat the Russians. Of course, it's so encrusted that I can't even get the yellow lid off. So, I get out an Exacto knife and cut a hole around the top. Since my blow torch is in the shop, I grab a pick-axe and slowly chip away at the chocolate crust, dying to taste the liquid gold that's inside. I know I'm a sight, but in my heart I also know I'm not alone. Whether it's chocolate syrup, coconut macaroons, or an entire case of Ding Dongs, we've all been there, haven't we?

Desperate, I run out to my car and grab the oil spout from the trunk. It's my only hope of getting to the chocolate, plus everybody knows that the faster you drink the syrup, the fewer calories you ingest. If I can just gulp it down quick enough, there's no way it will register on the log-in system that catalogues what goes in my mouth every day. (We've all told ourselves that one!) I lie on my kitchen floor, lifting the spout to my mouth, shoving it back in my throat, and hungrily gulping this can of artery clogger. When I get to the bottom, I toss it aside, spent. Satisfied, I stagger off to bed, hoping to fall back to sleep before the inevitable sugar migraine kicks in. Then I dream the dreams of the thin.

In my dreams, my thighs don't touch at the top. I know what color my pubic hair is. I can shave my legs without looking in the mirror. My profile no longer looks like Alfred Hitchcock's. The list goes on . . . .

If you share this dream, this book is for you. If you've ever thought about seeing your feet again, buying clothes in a single-digit size, or walking <u>down</u> a flight of stairs without getting winded, then you've come to the right place. This is a book for people who are tired of hearing a lot of New Age psychobabble about self-esteem and "changing eating habits forever."

This is the book for people who are tired of spending their hard-earned money on diets that just don't work. This is a book for people who eat so much they can't count high enough to add up all the calories they take in.

The Centers for Disease Control reports that there are 34 million fat people in America. Big deal. There are almost as many used-car salesmen, and no one's doing anything about them.

Do you know why there are so many fat people in America? Because they diet. And diets don't work.

I know because I've tried or know someone who's tried every one of them. There's Slim Fast, Weight Watchers, and Food Inhalers Anonymous. There's NutriSystem, Jenny Haag, and Arthur Murray. (The only support group I haven't joined is Save the Whales.) I tried liquid diets, diet pills, and my personal favorite— pancake batter and prune juice, better known as the Flap 'n' Crap Diet. I tried starvation, laxatives, and even vomiting. (Of course, that was only when I watched Susan Powter's infomercials!) I tried aerobicizing, *Sweating to the Oldies*, and the new Richard Simmons tape, *Collapsing to the Classics*. I tried lo-cal, no-cal, reduced-cal. Pretty much the only Cal I haven't tried is Ripken.

I even tried taping pictures to my refrigerator. Pictures of skinny women, pictures of fat women, and when I really wanted to kill my appetite, pictures of Wayne Newton.

We've all done it. Maybe not quite like me, but I know you've tried just about everything to stay thin: starvation, calorie-counting, and topping your food with spare parts from your kid's Legos. You've tried every diet under the sun, and then you found out what over 55 million other women discover every year: DIETS JUST DON'T WORK!

That's why 98 percent of all women gain all their weight back—and why 96 percent of them find a way to blame it on their husbands. Of course, those who don't gain the weight back—that lucky 2 percent—just look fabulous and live happily ever after. But who cares about skinny people? Television bombards us with pictures of skinny people. And while we all feel really bad about those starving people in Africa, there's not much we can do about it. Skinny people are not what this book is about. This is a book about fat people for fat people everywhere, and it's written by someone who really knows what it's like to be fat.

Susan Powter will tell you how to *Stop the Insanity* for $22.00. I can tell you how to lose weight in one sentence: Don't put anything in your mouth that gives you any satisfaction or pleasure whatsoever. But I know that's not what you want to hear. It's certainly not how I want to live. I like putting things in my mouth that make me feel good—that's how I ended up fat in the first place. And as soon as someone starts telling me I can't have those things, I do the very thing that you should also do: I tell them to stuff it, and then I start stuffing myself. So don't worry, you won't be getting any lessons in eating soybean paste from me.

When it comes to eating, there IS an alternative, but it's not very cost-effective. Oprah can eat all her favorite foods because she can afford to pay her personal nutritionist $58 million a year to figure out the top-secret formula for making French fries with no fat. (For my money, this has got to be the world's most valuable piece of information. If the United States Government had ever been able to come up with a way to make fat-free French fries, the Cold War would have ended a lot sooner). This might work for Oprah, but I don't have that kind of money. You probably don't either.

In the hundreds of attempts I've made to "start eating right," I've finally figured out what every woman in America already knows: IT COSTS TWICE AS MUCH MONEY TO EAT HEALTHY AS IT DOES TO PIG OUT. A bowl of blueberry muffin batter costs all of 93 cents and will last me a whole night! SKINLESS, BONELESS, TASTELESS chicken breasts are $4.00 a pound. "No-salt" spices are $3.50 a jar, and you're going to need about 83 of them to make your chicken edible.

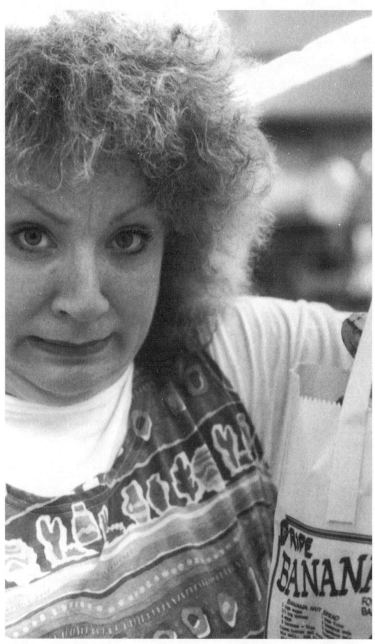

Nope. Not today.

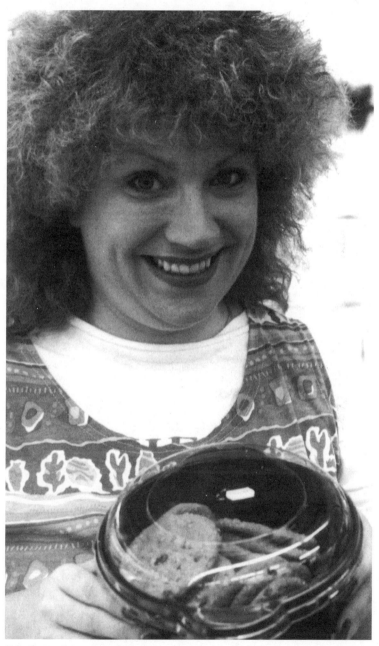

My favorite cereal.

Now, I'm not very good at math, but by my calculations, that's roughly $50,000 to eat something you hate. And when you can swing by KFC and get a three-piece dinner with mashy-tay-tays, baked beans, and two rolls for $3.49, it doesn't take a rocket scientist to figure out which way your wallet, not to mention your stomach, is going to go.

If you're like me, you don't want to DEAL your meals. You don't want to go to Jenny Haag and have your "counselor" regale you with the horrors of being ten pounds overweight and how she "overcame" it. PLEASE!!! Ten pounds overweight would be a blessing at this point. Jenny's ads say you can "Sign up now for just six cents a pound!" What they don't tell you is that you should cash in all your 401K savings if you want to be able to afford Jenny's "cuisine."

Is it just my TV, or is Jenny a little bit of a heifer herself? Maybe she should try gagging on her own Barf-o-Rama Beef Casserole every once in a while. Let her suffer like the rest of us!

And have you noticed that Weight Watchers meetings are always next to a TCBY store? Do they really think I want to sit around with other fat people and talk about all the things we love but will never be able to eat again? I tell you, every time I think I've found someone who really does understand, there's a catch. And we all know that nothing really understands our problems like an entire box of moon pies. That's why we drown our sorrows in them in the first place.

The thing is, I UNDERSTAND. I really do. I know what it means to be uncomfortable with the way you look. Right now, I weigh 230 pounds. But I know that somewhere in there, there's a 227-pound person trapped and trying to get out. Well, alright, maybe she's not trapped—I'm not saying it was a kidnapping or there's a ransom or anything. But I guarantee you that the 227-pound person is in there.

So you see, I've been there, and I'm here to tell you that I don't have the answer. I don't have one single answer for anybody but me. But what I do know is how it happened for me, how I dug myself to the bottom of a very long, deep hole but somehow made it back alive. So, hopefully, I can at least get you to the point of not feeling helpless. There's not one recipe in this book—except the ones I make fun of—and I'm not going to ask you to drag a slide rule down to the grocery store and do linear algebra every time you pick up a can of food.

It took me a lot of years to get to the point where I didn't HATE the idea of exercise and hate the idea of not getting as much as I wanted of everything I wanted every time I had something to eat. Because I was sure that there was an easier way that no one had discovered yet. And do you know what? In a way there was. But it was very painful and very difficult getting there. But it was also very, very necessary and just about the best thing I ever did for myself.

Don't worry, I'm not going to tell you it was worrying about my health that got me there. I know I'm not healthy, and I know I won't ever be. I smoke 500 cigarettes a day—that's after I cut off the filters—and I would rather be lying down than doing anything else.

I'm also not going to tell you to find an exercise you like. Guess what? If there were an exercise I liked, I wouldn't be fat! Don't you just love it when some so-called "weight-loss expert" goes down the list of exercises for you, like she's convinced that there MUST be one that you just haven't thought of yet?

"What about a walk in the park?"

"I hate the park."

"How about tennis?"

"Excuse me?! Oh my God! I FORGOT ALL ABOUT TENNIS! I LOVE TENNIS! I LOVE darting back and forth at upwards of three miles per hour, looking like a complete moron, with so much sweat pouring off my body so fast that salmon are trying to swim upstream to spawn."

Let me tell you how I feel about exercise. If I'm putting on earrings (three calories), and I drop the back of one on the floor, I'll change to a different pair just to avoid bending over to pick the damn thing up. That's how much effort I like to exert, so I don't think tennis is going to solve my problems. So, shut up!

None of this garbage is going to solve your problems, but it can be done. I'm not saying you're ever going to be as thin as you want or as happy as you want, but you know what? It doesn't matter. You can keep throwing good money after bad, trying to discover the skinny neurotic person inside you. Or you can just give up and save the $23,000 the average American spends on weight loss every year.

So grab a box of Twinkies and a nice creamy milkshake, curl up on the couch, and sit back and read my story. You'll laugh, you'll cry (but only because some of the jokes are so bad), and you might just learn a thing or two, such as how to tell if you have a weight problem, where to shop for fat clothes, and all about the two diets that really do work.

And as you listen to my story, you're probably going to hear your story as well. If you don't, then I'm probably not shouting loud enough. But don't worry, I can always scream louder.

Remember, I'm not angry.

I'm hungry!

PART ONE

Getting Fat

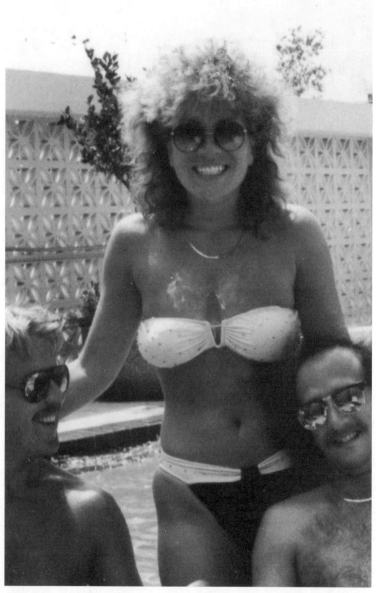

The good ol' days. By the way, that's suntan lotion on my chest.

ONE

Tipping the Scales

The first thing you do when you're fat is change your hair color. You think you will look better, but you just look fat with a different hair color.

Believe it or not, I wasn't always this BIG. (Not that many kids weigh 230 pounds when they're born). I actually looked pretty good until about three years ago. But then my life really took a downward spiral. If you've ever been through one of these periods (once a month!), then you probably know what I'm talking about. You're so depressed that you can't get out of bed. All you can do is sit there and stuff your face, and before you know it, you're too fat to get out of bed. Before you know it, you look up and three or four days have gone by, and you've put on 100 pounds. I believe the clinical term for this behavior is being a fat, lazy pig.

When I look back now, it's easy to see what happened to me (hindsight is 20/20 and about 125 pounds lighter). First of all, I turned 30, so I figured I got a free 25 pounds just for that. That took me up to about 165. Then the only man I ever really loved—other than Chef Boyardee—left me, which meant I had no choice but to put on another 25 pounds. Now I'm up to 190 and really bummed out. So there's only one thing to do: go see my shrink. BIG mistake. That's how I got up to 230 pounds.

My therapist, God bless her, is an understanding woman (Lord knows, she should be after seventeen years and $250,000), so she did exactly what I wanted her to do—she wrote me a prescription. The only problem was, the prescription wasn't for anything fun, and it didn't have a high street value, like methadone. It was for an ANTIDEPRESSANT, and I think you know what that means.

I've taken a lot of antidepressants over the last 17 years, so I know what they do. They make me—and you—gain weight. Recently they've come out with new antidepressants, like Prozac and Paxil, that don't make you put on the pounds. I once tried Prozac for a couple of weeks and gunned down three people at Kiddie Pizza Place. So I guess I'm one of the unlucky few who can't take these miracles of modern medicine and have my soul saved.

The point is, I have to take the old trycyclic antidepressants, and guess what their number-one side effect is? WEIGHT GAIN!! So basically what happened was, I went to the shrink because I was depressed about being fat, and she gave me pills that make me even fatter. It's a vicious cycle: I schedule another appointment, go in, and talk about how depressed I am over getting fatter. Then the doctor renews my prescription for more pills to make me fatter still.

If you want to know a big secret, listen up: PROZAC DOESN'T KEEP YOU FROM GAINING WEIGHT! The doctors just figure that if you're not depressed, you won't eat as much. WRONG!! If you truly love food— and who doesn't?—Prozac won't make a dent in your appetite. In other words, all this stuff about Prozac not causing weight gains is A LIE, so don't run out and ask for a prescription. (By the way, if you do get a Prozac prescription, each pill costs $88, which comes to $32,120 each year.)

THE DECLINE

I always say that G. was the love of my life. Everyone agrees that when I met him I was the healthiest I've ever been (when I say everyone, I mean me, my mother, my friends, and the bathroom scale). I LOOKED spectacular, I was in great shape emotionally, and boy was I ready for him. Not only does G. have one of the best reputations in the comedy business, but he's also the nicest guy you'll ever meet.

Oddly enough, the first time I met G., I was dating someone else. That guy was the most emotionally under-developed child I had ever met. So I naturally thought G. was the weirdo because he was so nice. He didn't cheat on his girlfriend, he didn't smoke or drink, and he'd never done time.

Two years later, after Peter Pan dumped me, I ran into G. again. I don't know what had happened to me, but I was at long last ready to meet a nice guy. (Actually, I do know what had happened to me— I was sick of dating psychos.) But I never thought that nice guy would be G. He wasn't my type physically, but then we got stuck working together for a week. The more time I spent with him, the more I became attracted to him, and at the end of the week, I was in love.

The miracle was, he loved me back! I didn't know if I deserved it, but I didn't really care. All of a sudden, I knew that every bad thing that had happened to me in my life was okay and worth the suffering, because God had brought me G. And for a long time, everything was great. All we did was laugh. Never before and never since has ANYONE made me laugh like G. did. There was only one problem: ME.

As it turned out, it hadn't been that hard to attract G. in the first place. The whole thing happened so easily and naturally, that in a strange way, even though it was great, I guess I took it for granted. For some stupid reason, I didn't realize that once I HAD G., there were still certain things that I had to do to KEEP him. Looking back, it all seems so obvious, but it sure wasn't at the

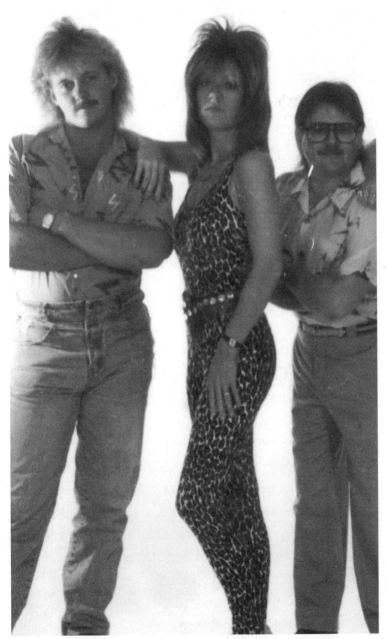

Nice tiger suit! Nice wig! But, God, look at my ARMS!

time. And when you're in a relationship and not holding up your end of the bargain, that's a very BIG problem. Pretty soon, so was I.

Very slowly, I started packing on the pounds. Kind of like Grecian formula, it was slow and gradual, and I almost didn't even notice. It's amazing how you can tell yourself that the reason your jeans don't fit anymore is because they're shrinking in the dryer, not because you're turning into a wide load.

Then I started to smoke again. I guess I thought the cigarettes would help me keep the pounds off, but I was wrong. Pretty soon, I wasn't looking so good. By the time two years had passed, I had let myself go—BIG TIME! Before I knew it, I looked like Luciano Pavarotti in drag. The only problem was, I didn't have two Grammys on the TV in the den and a couple billion dollars in the bank. But other than that, we were identical—at least, that's how I remember it.

Saint that he was, G. tried to help me. My God he tried, but let's face it, if you don't want to take care of yourself, there's not much that anyone can do to get you to do otherwise. G. drove me to every shrink, paid for every diet, encouraged me, and even loved me unconditionally. But it wasn't enough. As it turned out, nothing short of every French fry in America would have been enough. So after much begging, pleading, and hiding the baked goods, G. finally had enough. Long past the point that any other human would have been able to endure me, he finally had to leave.

Looking back, I don't blame him—but somehow my appetite still does.

Naturally, I reacted to his departure as any other normal, red-blooded, desperate, neurotic, insane woman with screwed-up hormones, no metabolism, and an out-of-control appetite would. I started drinking heavily and eating my way into oblivion. Pretty soon my bedroom floor was covered in candy wrappers, pizza boxes, fast-food garbage, and empty bottles of booze. It wasn't a pretty sight, especially after the trash got high enough that it actually became a PART of my bed. My room looked like an outtake from *Who's Afraid of Virginia Woolf?*

The worst part of it was that I didn't leave the house for something like six months. I started to look like a vampire. I never saw the light of day, so my skin turned all pasty and white. My skin was so unhealthy that you could have seen through it if it weren't for all that fat underneath. The few times that I did venture outside my cave—pretty much only at night—I would run into people who hadn't seen me in a couple of years, and their eyes would get HUGE. They couldn't believe it was me. Neither could I.

There is a moral to this story. It took me a long time to recognize it, and it's probably one of those things that you'll never understand until you've gone through it yourself, but I learned that EVEN THE GREATEST LOVE CANNOT KEEP YOU FROM DESTROYING YOURSELF. I know those of you that have never been

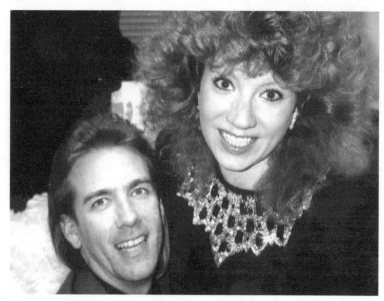

The one that got away.

through this are laughing right now and saying, "Yeah, sure, Beth. We've heard it all before." And you're right. But let me tell you, if you've been through something like this, then you know what I'm talking about. And if you haven't . . . well, just pray to God that you never have to. It cost me my greatest love.

THAT'S WHAT FRIENDS ARE FOR

The whole time I was going through my own personal hell, my best friend Brian tried to help me through it. Now, if you've ever watched anyone suffer through a horrible funk like this, you probably know you pretty much have to let them suffer through it on their own. Much as you'd like to help, the best thing you can do is

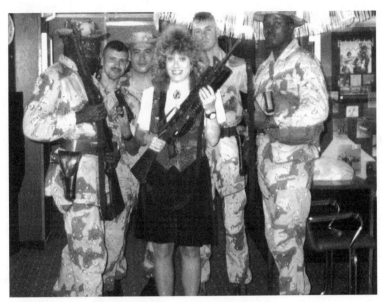

Goin' to catch some vittles in Saudi Arabia.

stay out of their way and let them bottom out on their own.

It's sort of like watching a plane crash: You see that something horrible is about to happen, but you can't run out there and catch the damn thing. You just have to let that 747 wide-body fall to the ground. Once it hits, you can check for survivors. At the very least, you can forage for a WHOLE LOT of free honey-roasted peanuts. And when I talk about 747 wide-bodies, that's exactly what I looked like in those days. I needed a full ground crew just to get me ready to leave the hangar—er, house—in the morning.

So even though there really wasn't anything he could do for me, Brian also tried. To give me some idea of how big I'd become, he gave me hints all the time. But I just wasn't listening. Or maybe I wasn't ready to hear. I don't know which it was, but the bottom line is, I was in BIG TROUBLE. So was my butt.

At some point, in the midst of all this, Brian and I took a trip to Hawaii. I was so fed up with life and so embarrassed about how I looked, that the last thing I wanted to do was go outside. (Actually, I pretty much hate being outside to begin with, so this was really nothing new. But trust me, I was not doing well.) Even though I was surrounded by some of the most spectacular geography known to man—A MAN WHO LOOKS GOOD IN A BATHING SUIT, that is—all I wanted to do was tour the souvenir shops.

Brian put up with all of this, but he also brought along a camera so he could videotape me wherever we went. While the film was rolling, he kept up a running commentary about how I was the only person in the universe who didn't want to see Hawaii. Meanwhile, I spent all day, every day looking at all these fascinating little Hawaiian key chains with the islands' different gods on them. For instance, there's the god of happiness (not me), the god of peace (again, not me), and the god of health (definitely not me). Finally I found a key chain with a god I'd never seen before. I turned to Brian and said, "Look, it's the god of diet!"

All Brian could say was, "You've certainly angered him!"

True story. And to this day, I absolutely LOVE the tape of that trip. It's great to have a video chronicle of the depths to which you've sunk in your life, if for no other reason than you'll always know how far you've come. As for Brian, he could not have been a better friend. He stuck with me during a period when the chips were really down—my throat, that is, with plenty of salsa to boot.

Now, the moral of this story is not that you should get really fat and photograph yourself at your worst. Sure, there are a good number of porno magazines that would gladly print those pictures, but that's not good for your self-image. No, the moral is that no matter how heavy you get, you DEFINITELY have to maintain your sense of humor about things. There's no better way to get through life. That's what this book is all about. Of course, it also helps if you have a friend like Brian. He's the best.

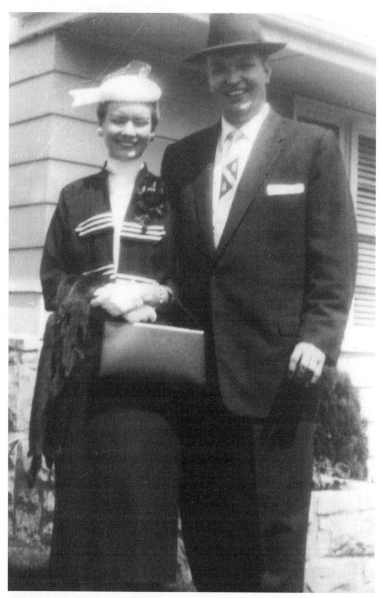

Mom and Dad, 1955. Full of hope. Little did they know in seven years, they would be the parents of a psychotic, co-dependent food addict.

TWO

This Is All My Parents' Fault...Isn't It?

On Halloween, my Dad always had to "test" our candy.
That's the only reason I want to have children.

This is all my parents' fault, isn't it?

I must have had some near-death experience with fruit as a child. To this day, I can't bear to look at it, be near it, smell it, let alone think about eating it. I don't like anything about it, especially not the taste. You're not going to believe this—well, okay, you've seen the pictures; maybe you do believe me—but I have never eaten a banana—they're just too squishy. Of course, not being a fruit lover, or even fruit tolerator, you can imagine how hard it is to lose weight when pretty much EVERY diet known to woman begins and ends with fruit. The only saving grace is that it's kept me from getting stuck on one of those all-fruit diets, the kind where you lose 50 pounds in a week because all you do is sit on the can for seven straight days.

Have I mentioned that I also hate vegetables, chicken, fish, and water? I don't remember eating any of this stuff as a kid, and my taste buds stopped taking applications after age three—the strained-beef incident (don't ask). Dad, of course, couldn't have cared less. He would have been perfectly happy with a vending machine in the kitchen. And while my mom is a wonderful woman, I don't think healthy food was something she had heard of. In fact, I think she was better at balancing her checkbook than balancing our diets.

With a background like this, I think you can imagine what my eating habits were like when I was a kid. All you need to know about healthy food in our house is

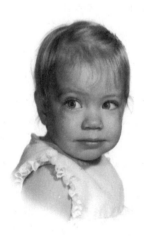

The one and only time you'll see me in a sleeveless dress.

that there wasn't any. Actually, let me correct that. I vaguely recall a bowl of little, round green things—perhaps they were peas, I don't really know—going totally unnoticed and untouched in the center of our kitchen table. I think they were there through most of the Nixon presidency.

So listen to me, people: I didn't want fruit then, and I don't want it now. So I'm sure as hell not going to pay any attention to any diet that tells me I'm going to have to eat a lot of it. I'm sick and tired of people trying to jam fruits and veggies down my throat.

In school, no one ever got in trouble for having celery in their desk. It was always candy and gum.

GYM CLASS

When I was a kid I would do anything to get out of gym class. In high school I told all my teachers I had leukemia and that gym was the only hour when I could go to chemotherapy. I'm ashamed of that now, but at 15 it seemed like a good excuse. I hated that class more than anything, and I still think it should be outlawed. If you don't like to run around and sweat by the seventh grade, then three years of flag football aren't going to change your mind. I was ALWAYS the last person picked for ANY team. Except when we had a tug of war. Then every team wanted me for their anchor.

Oddly enough, I was on the swim team for a couple of years. I HATED it, but it was what all the popular girls were doing, so I did it just to try to fit in. I was ALWAYS the last one to finish every race. The lights in the pool would be out and the coach would be sleeping in a corner. (You can't really blame him for napping at 11:00 P.M.) I hated every minute of it, and it didn't make me any more popular. I just got hungrier.

To this day, I can't stand swimming—and not just because I can't find a flattering bathing suit. It's because inevitably you have to get out of the water, and believe me, I do not look good wet—I look like *The Creature from the Black Lagoon.*

MY FIRST DIET

Of course, I wasn't always fat. So the first time I tried dieting it wasn't even intentional. Back in high school, I wasn't even remotely heavy—this was the seventies, so I think my hairstyle weighed even more than I did. (Lord knows, my hair has tried to keep up with my body weight through the years, but somewhere along the way, even though my hair got bigger, the body weight won out.)

As I said, that first diet—speed and vodka—wasn't even meant to be one. I started taking the speed to stay awake during class, and speed being speed, soon enough I was taking it just to GET AWAKE in the morning. BAD IDEA! Nuts at the time, I decided I really liked speed for three reasons:

1. I was in high school, so I felt like it was "cool" to take it.

2. Since it made social studies go by a whole lot faster, it made social studies a lot more interesting.
3. I never gained weight.

As for the vodka, well, it was the seventies, and that's what they were serving in the cafeteria. So there it is, my first diet: speed and vodka. Speed to wake up, vodka to go to sleep, and no food in between—a diet I'm pretty sure wouldn't get FDA approval today. Plus, speed makes you grind your teeth and kill people. But come to think of it, most other diets do that anyway. And in the long run, it just doesn't work. Ask Elvis! Well, I guess you can't.

Bear in mind, I AM NOT ADVOCATING DRUG USE! It's just that I was a stupid, reckless, rebellious teenager. Actually, there was one other problem with this method: I didn't need to diet. I wasn't fat in high school, but I sure thought I was. Back then, I was just a skinny little strung-out string bean (that's what speed and vodka will do to you) who wished she would grow up and have lots of curves, just like a real woman. I guess my wish came true—and then some. But growing up in this twisted, sick culture of ours will convince a woman that she needs to lose a few pounds even though what she really needs to do is get off the speed and vodka.

I think every girl in my high school class was worried about her weight—the vomiting in the girls' room was regular enough that the school band could practice to it. And they did. You should have heard the school fight song; it was rewritten to include a chorus where the whole student body stuck their fingers down their throats in unison. The football team won the state championship that year: no other school wanted to play us. No wonder they changed the school colors to yellow and green.

PART TWO

Being Fat

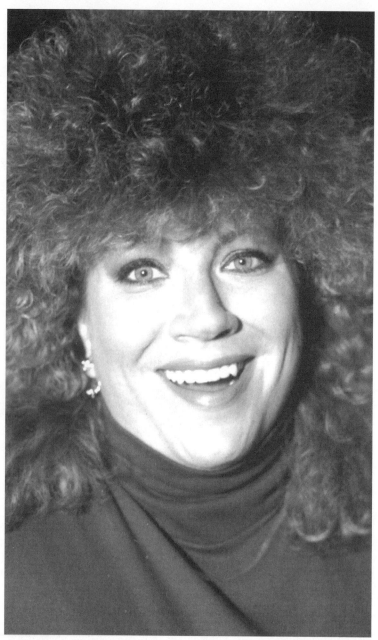

The biggest human head known to man!

THREE

You Know You're Fat When...

I was at McDonald's the other day, and the drive-through line took FOREVER. When I got to the window, the guy handed me my food and said, "Sorry about the wait." I thought he said, "Sorry about the weight," so I replied, "Sorry you're still wearing a name tag at 33."

Most of us can tell we're way too fat just by looking in the mirror. For instance, if all of you won't fit in the mirror, it's a pretty good indication that you could stand to lose a pound or two. Or, if the mirror you're using looks like a fun-house mirror at the carnival, but you actually bought the damn thing at Harold's House of Crap, then you're probably carrying some extra baggage that needs to be checked at the gate before you board the flight that is the rest of your life. And if flight attendants tell you that you'll have to check yourself, then you know exactly what I'm talking about. But don't worry, you've come to the right place.

For those of you who are still in denial, those of you who aren't really sure if you're overweight, here's a simple test you can use to evaluate the status of your own weight problem:

You know you're fat when . . .

1. You go to an all-you-can-eat buffet and the manager has a bouncer watching you.
2. Your idea of dinner conversation is, "Who wants fourths?"
3. You read *USA Today* just to see the pie charts.
4. Domino's is calling YOU.
5. You qualify for a loan from Greenpeace.
6. You need a shoe horn to get into an airplane seat.
7. You go on a whale-watching trip and everyone on the boat has their cameras pointed at you.
8. Your boyfriend breaks up with you because he says he's "under too much pressure"... because you like to make love on top.
9. You get an invitation to be in the Macy's Thanksgiving Day parade—as a FLOAT.
10. You walk into a restaurant alone and the hostess still asks, "How many in your party?"
11. You go to put on your seat belt and it only goes as far as your navel.
12. You get on an elevator and four people volunteer to get off.

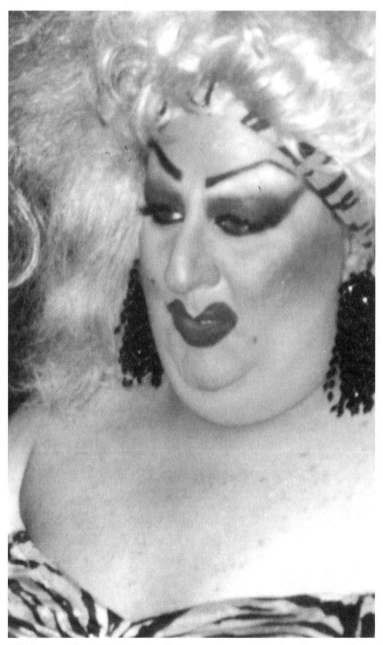

Me when I'm 50 (okay, 35).

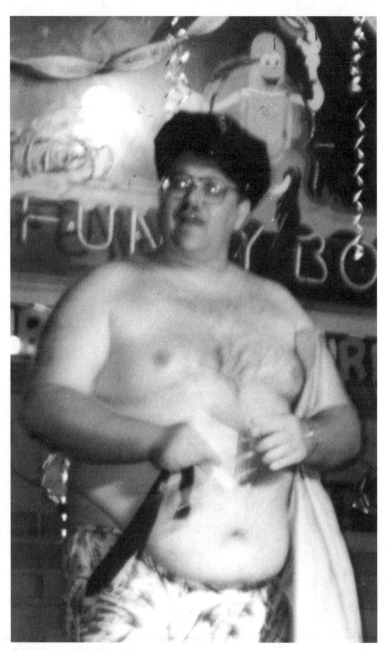

My future husband.

SCORING: If even one of these statements applies to you, then the bad news is that you definitely have a weight problem. If none of these statements apply to you, then WHY ARE YOU READING THIS BOOK?

If you're still not sure whether this book is for you, a few more diagnostic scenarios follow that you may want to consider. This is the long-answer portion of the test, so see if any of the following apply to you:

YOU PROBABLY HAVE A WEIGHT PROBLEM IF . . .

1. YOU FAIL CERTAIN TESTS.

For example, you try to pinch an inch and end up getting out your husband's tape measure that stretches out to eight feet. You also know you're in trouble if pinching an inch sets off a ripple of shock waves that can be measured on the Richter scale.

2. FOOD IS A PRIORITY IN YOUR LIFE.

I'll never forget the most insane thing I ever did. After getting suitably plastered at a bar one night, I was making my nightly drive past my ex-boyfriend's house to look for strange cars in his driveway. It was pouring down rain, and my windshield wipers stopped working. Naturally, I decided to speed up. I don't know why I thought it was so important to speed by his house; it's not like he was sitting in his window at 4:00 A.M. hoping I would drive by. So there I was in the middle of the night, speeding through the driving rain with no windshield wipers. Great idea!

Since no one in his right mind was out and about at that hour (except other drunk, stupid women driving past their exes' houses), and there weren't any moving targets for me to hit, I chose a stationary one. I PLOWED into a parked car and slammed it up over the curb and into someone's front yard. (Warning: Drinking and driving don't mix, so don't try this with your own car. Use a friend's.)

Normally in a situation like this, I would do the right thing; stop and leave a note with someone else's name and address on it. But since Hardee's was due to close in half an hour, I didn't have enough time for formalities. So even though the hood of my car was up over my windshield and twisted into a weird, accordion shape, I skipped the note and rushed straight to Hardee's. I went through the drive-through, ate my food, and then went back to leave a note.

You can imagine how surprised the car's owners were the next morning when they went out, saw the note, and called the telephone number on it, only to get a recording telling them that Domino's wasn't open yet. The moral of this story: Always remember the phone number of the nearest pizza place.

3. YOUR LEGS ARE SO POCKMARKED, THEY LOOK LIKE YOU GOT SHOT WITH A ROUND OF BBs.

I'll never forget the day I realized I had cellulite. I

was in the shower, shaving my thighs (it was Easter), and my razor popped a wheelie! Those were some big bumps, kids. Of course, the cellulite isn't as bad as the big wad of fat behind each of my knees. (What the hell is <u>that</u>? And are they related to the ones under my armpits?) Not real attractive, folks. Plus, there is absolutely NO WAY to sit without them showing, especially in the car. When I used to be able to fold one leg under the other, I would try hiding the fat that way. (It makes it kind of tough to drive a stick shift, let me tell you.) It would STILL jump out like that little Pop-N-Fresh Biscuits guy. (The Pillsbury people thought they were his long-lost brothers, and for a while there, my knees almost had a three-commercial deal.)

4. CERTAIN ACTIVITIES BECOME DIFFICULT, SUCH AS:

<u>GETTING OUT OF THE CAR</u>. I have to rock three times just to get enough momentum going before I summon the strength to hurl myself out onto the street. I won't even tell you about the sound the seat makes when I do this, but suffice to say, it's not very attractive on a date. Come to think of it, it pretty much grosses me out when I'm ALONE.

<u>PAINTING YOUR TOENAILS</u>. I have very pretty feet. Long ago, when I used to be able to reach my toenails, I would paint them every week. Now I have to grip the paintbrush between a pair of chopsticks. My toes end up looking like I painted them with a roller.

When I get the money, I'm going to switch to a Wagner Power Painter.

GETTING OUT OF THE BATHTUB. This story is going to sound ridiculous, but I swear it's completely true. Being in the stand-up comedy business means I travel A LOT and stay in hotels all over the place. Because I don't trust hotel bathtubs when I'm on the road, I only use the shower. So when I'm home for a couple of days, a nice long, luxurious bath is my big treat. (Warning: The following sentence is for women only; if any guys are reading this, please skip it for your own safety.) This will come as a surprise to some of you, but I have a real girlie bathroom, full of special oils, bubbles, and crystals, as well as positive affirmation tapes and angels—but I swear, absolutely NO PICTURES OF DAVID HASSELHOFF. (Guys, you can start reading again.)

I'd returned from the road and I was lying there in the bath. My three hours were up, so I went ahead and let the water out. The only problem was, I guess my butt had gotten a little bigger since the last time I'd been home. I guess when submerged in hot water, my butt swelled a bit, because I had created a form-fitting, hermetically sealed, gravity-defying DAM in my tub, so I thought that all the water had drained from the tub. But when I stood up—WHOOSH! Gallon upon gallon of water went barreling down the tub towards the drain.

It was bad enough that my bathroom suddenly looked like one of those Wet-N-Wild amusement parks

(I just stood there swirling toward the drain while cling-ing to my little blue bath mat for dear life), but imagine my surprise when three neighborhood kids turned up riding the waves on their rafts! Then the little rats had the gall to ask if they could go on the ride again. I charged each one $15 for the whole afternoon. Easiest money I ever made.

Any of this sound familiar? I know it does. So keep reading.

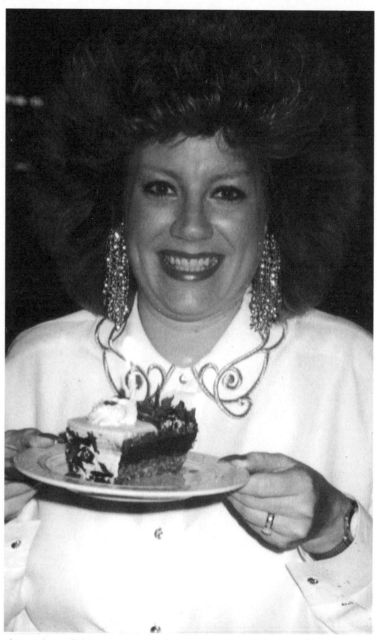

Appetizer first.

FOUR

Eating Wrong

My four favorite words are "All You Can Eat."

When it comes to food, the bottom line is, I HATE TO FEEL DEPRIVED! I would rather eat one contact lens full of chili than 5,000 grapes. And if one more person says to me, "How can you not like FRUIT?" I swear I'm going to punch them. I DON'T KNOW WHY I DON'T LIKE FRUIT! I JUST DON'T!

You hear a lot of stuff about fruit these days. But of course, the thing you REALLY hear about all the time is FAT. "You must get rid of the fat in your diet," they say. "And you must do it now!" Well guess what, kids? I love fat! I love everything fat is in. Even though you can't see it or smell it, I know in one second if it's not there. And I want it in my life—I just don't want it on my butt. Therein lies my dilemma. And the bad news is, I don't know the answer. All I know is that if I want a decent-looking guy, a successful career, and a steady heartbeat, I have to stop eating everything I love.

There are a lot of diets that will tell you, "Oh, you CAN have all of those things, just not as MUCH." THAT'S A LIE. Well, "not as much" to them just won't fill my fingernail and then I feel DEPRIVED (even with my fingernails, which are long enough to pick my nose from another area code). Basically, people who talk about "eating what you want" are lying to you, because "eating what I want" means EATING HOW <u>MUCH</u> I WANT. NOT AS MUCH AS YOU'RE WILLING TO <u>LET ME HAVE</u>.

EATING OUT

When most people diet, they spend way too much time worrying about what's going to happen to their self-control when they eat at a restaurant. The people at Jenny Haag, for example, make a real big deal out of this topic, as if you're suddenly going to panic and order everything on the menu.

Panicking about eating out when you're dieting really bugs me, and not just because it assumes that you don't have enough self-control to contain your own appetite and urges. (You don't!) No, the reason it really makes me mad is because there's nothing I love more than going out to eat. The whole point of the experience is to stuff your face with food that you normally wouldn't prepare for yourself. Believe me, if I could I'd set up Big Boy's All-You-Can-Eat Barbecue Bar in my kitchen.

But I can't, and that's the reason I go to Big Boy's in the first place. I don't go there for the decor or beauty tips from the waitresses.

The other people who take all the fun out of going to a restaurant are the morons who can't ever seem to order food the way it's supposed to be eaten. For instance, there is nothing in the world that pisses me off more than going out to eat with someone you THOUGHT was your friend and listening to them order their salad dressing <u>ON THE SIDE</u>. Sorry,

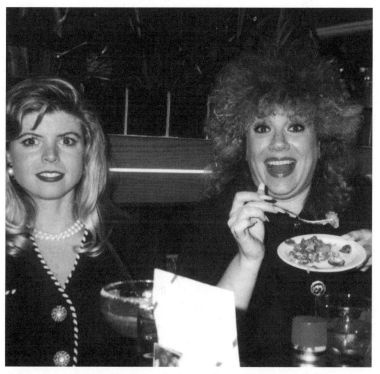

After zapping my sister-in-law, Laura Lyn, with a stun-gun, I steal her dessert!

friends, but nothing should EVER be ordered on the side—with the possible exception of jalapeño peppers or extra gravy.

When it comes to restaurants in this great country of ours, no one knows them like my good friend Tom Sobel. He runs a booking agency in Louisville, Kentucky, and one of the reasons I love working for him is that he knows the best places to eat in almost every city in the United States. I always tell him, "I don't care how far I have to drive, just book me around the great restaurants." And if he's able, he'll book a tour around them for me.

Tom turned me on to a great place in New York City, a sushi automat at 34th Street and 5th Avenue. Kind of a strange idea, I know, but trust me, it's worth the trip. The restaurant has a racetrack-shaped lunch counter and a big circular chain-link belt that goes around with food on it. All the dishes are priced according to the color of the plate, so when you're finished eating, you just bring your plates up to the cashier, and she adds them up for you. My God, it was so much fun, I even forgot that I hate sushi! That revolving racetrack was entertaining enough to get me to eat raw fish!

If you're ever in Los Angeles, Tom recommends a place called Oki-Dog. Brace yourself, because this is going to sound a little weird. An Oki-Dog is served in a flour tortilla; it's two hot dogs wrapped in pastrami and covered with chili, cheese, and onions. Trust me, it's delicious. And if you're there, be sure to try the fresh-squeezed orange juice. (Fresh fruit's close kin, I know, but the juice is far more palatable.)

Here's one I haven't tried, but Tom swears by it and it sounds legendary—in Owensboro, Kentucky, a restaurant called The Moonlight Inn that will barbecue ANYTHING. Chicken, pork, beef, mutton, lamb, fish, car seats, lizard purses, you name it. Just bring it in, and they'll grill it up for you. The late, great comedians Zack and Mack once ate 18 pounds of ribs there—AND THAT WAS JUST THEIR APPETIZER. I hope to personally break their record if I'm ever in the neighborhood.

DON'T FORGET

One of my all-time favorite lines has to be, "Oh, gosh, I forgot to eat." Don't you just love people who say that? I find the concept completely mind-boggling. I mean, FORGETTING to eat? Really. I can understanding forgetting to shower, forgetting to brush your teeth, forgetting to go to work, forgetting to get dressed, and forgetting to go to the bathroom when you have to pee in the middle of the night. But forgetting to EAT? How can anyone forget the one thing that swirls through our minds on an endless loop 24 hours a day, 365 days a year? I tell you what, folks, WHENEVER I'm eating, I'm already planning my next meal. Forget all this "live in the moment" crap. I say, LIVE IN YOUR NEXT MEAL—if it has a lot of gravy, you can even bathe in it. There's no better place to be. Live in the future.

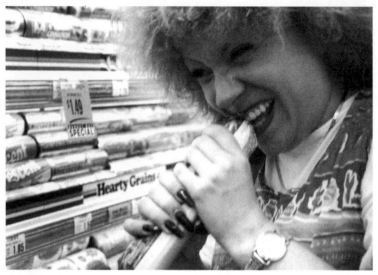

Cookie time!

MY FAVORITE FOODS

I love making chocolate chip cookies, but the problem is, by the time I've finished eating the dough, there's usually not enough left to make more than five cookies. And buying cookie dough already made in the tube doesn't work either. Isn't it amazing how easily the stuff glides down your throat? That wrapping paper just peels off those rolls of dough like a banana skin, and that's as close as I get to fruit.

What really cracks me up is Chocolate Chip Cookie Dough ice cream. Is this supposed to somehow <u>seem</u> like the dough is HEALTHIER for you just because it's mixed in with the richest vanilla ice cream on the planet? Still, we all run to the stores like a herd of buffalo for the stuff, don't we? As far as I'm concerned, however, the ice cream only gets in the way—which means I have to go on a scavenger hunt for the little nuggets of cookie dough. Of course, they only put about two of them in the entire pint of ice cream, and I can't afford to rent a back-hoe to find the treasured, sacred scraps of the stuff. Thanks a lot guys. I think I'll stick with the real thing.

Wedding cake is one of my all-time favorite foods. I love it, and I crash weddings all the time just to get some. You probably don't realize it, but sleeping with a piece of wedding cake under your pillow really DOES bring you good luck. For example, you just won't believe how lucky you feel when you wake up in the middle of the night and YOU DON'T EVEN HAVE TO GET OUT OF BED TO GET CAKE!

You can imagine how fed up I am with going to yuppie weddings and dealing with this hideous new trend of "healthy" wedding cakes. As far as I'm concerned, there's no point in going to the damn wedding if you're not even going to get something good to eat. Screw romance.

You know the story: You're at the wedding and you spot it in the corner the second you get to the reception. (It's the only reason you made the trip to begin with.) It's five feet tall, white, and COVERED with the coveted white sugar roses. You fight your way to the front of the line. (Let some other desperate bridesmaid catch the bouquet; you're here for the cake.) You get your wedge, you bite in, AND IT'S TOFU! To add insult to injury, they tell you the roses are real flowers, because "We care about our guests' health." Please! If you really cared about health and well-being, you'd care about the bride's health and you wouldn't have put real flowers on tofu, because now I'm going to have to punch her out.

Well, that's enough of this topic. I'm starved.

The Genie appears and says, "Beth, you have three wishes."

"No problem," I reply. "Gravy, rolls, and butter."

FOOD TIPS

• IF YOU ABSOLUTELY <u>MUST</u> ORDER PIZZA, EAT HALF OF IT AND THEN DUMP YOUR ASHTRAY ON THE OTHER HALF <u>BEFORE</u> YOU THROW IT IN THE GARBAGE. That way, when you go to dig it out at 4:00 A.M., you won't be able to eat it. Okay, I admit you can still eat it, but I don't advise it. The heartburn is UNBELIEVABLE—trust me, I've tried it. Several times.

If you don't smoke, try drowning the pizza in dishwashing liquid. There is NO WAY you can eat a pizza covered in soap. I promise. (I recommend Dawn for this job. Then, if you decide you <u>still</u> have to eat the damn thing, Dawn will "take grease out of your gut," just like the commercial says.)

• IF YOU BUY A GALLON OF ICE CREAM, EAT HALF OF IT. Then set the container in the sink filled halfway with hot water. The second, THE VERY

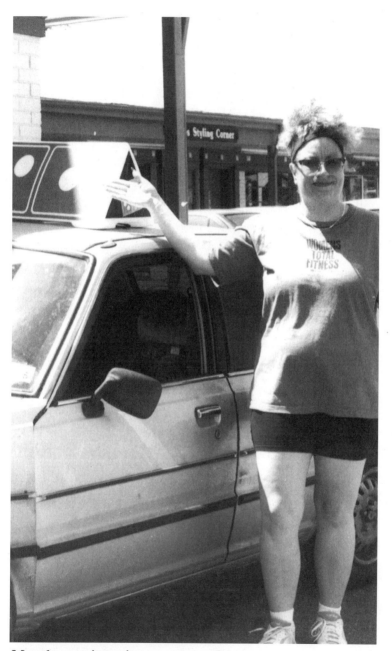

My other car's an ice cream truck.

INSTANT it melts, pour it down the drain. The best thing about this trick is that I've never known anyone to successfully get down the drain after melted ice cream—our arms are just too fat.

• DON'T BUY STUFF AT THE GROCERY STORE THAT YOU KNOW YOU'RE NEVER GOING TO EAT. Don't kid yourself. For example, pineapple. When I was in Hawaii, I loved it floating in a giant flaming Mai Tai. I will eat through fire AND fruit to get to the liquor, but the pineapple just doesn't taste the same when you get it at the local supermarket. If you're going to waste money, waste it on something you love. Buy all your favorite foods, eat half, drown them in dishwashing detergent, and toss 'em.

• FORGET PASTA. There's a rumor going around that it's good for you. It is. But only if you drown it in enough butter, mozzarella, and Reese's Pieces to give it flavor. That's the catch. There's ALWAYS a catch.

• STAY AWAY FROM DIETS THAT PROMISE, "YOU CAN STILL EAT ALL OF YOUR FAVORITE FOODS!" Lies! First of all, you're doing that already, so if that were really true, you'd be thin as a rail. Which brings me to my second point. If the diet says you can still eat all your favorite foods, you CAN, but only once a year with an armed guard at your side counting your three teaspoonsful.

• AVOID THE FOOD PYRAMID AT ALL COSTS. I'm really sick and tired of all these barf-foods that the government now says we're supposed to eat six times a day. (These are the same people who used to tell us to eat plenty of red meat and dairy products, remember?)

Take grains—please. Have you ever had a piece of 12-GRAIN bread? I swear to you, it tastes just like boogers—not that I've ever eaten boogers. (At least not since I started going to Boogers Anonymous six years ago.) What I mean is, this bread tastes like what I think boogers taste like. You bite into a piece of this 12-grain bread, and you're just chewing along, minding your own business and thinking about your next meal, and BAM! You squish down on what they want you to believe is a piece of grain, but you and I both know what it really is: A BOOGER! Would someone please tell me what kind of grain is squishy? And then, there's bran. I'd like to choke whoever discovered bran.

• EAT REAL FOOD. Stay away from anything that people try to convince you is food, but your taste buds know isn't. Examples include tofu, seaweed, all health foods, and any one-calorie frozen "yogurt" that is really made out of a space-age polymer.

In order to obey this commandment, I do most of my eating at convenience stores, especially when I'm on the road. Believe me, they have nothing but REAL food at convenience stores: nachos, chili dogs, chips, dips, and, of course, all your favorite offerings from Hostess and Tasty Cake. I once spent $117 at a 7–Eleven. Do you know how hungry you have to be to spend $117 at a 7–Eleven?

In fact, the only thing worse than these disgusting, so-called healthy excuses for foods are the people who have been eating them all along. (Yes, California, that means you.)

• ALWAYS LOOK FOR FREE FOOD. Happy hours are a great place to get free food. Buy a drink and then meander over to the buffet. You can go through five or six times before they catch you and throw you out. I also recommend eating contests. At chili cook-offs, you're EXPECTED to eat 500 bowls of chili. For dessert, try the pie-eating contest!

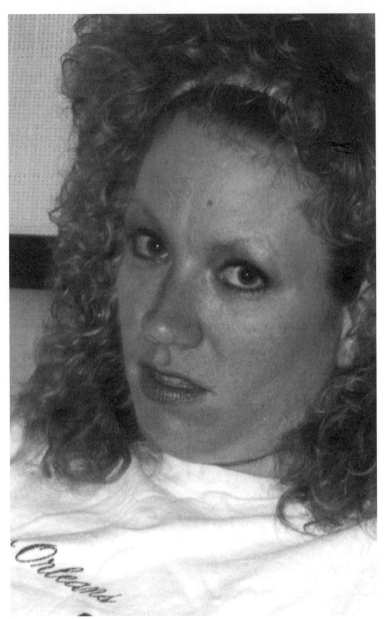

It's been 31 minutes. Call Domino's and see what the holdup is!

FIVE

I Never Met a Diet I Liked

I always tell people I'm eating for two. I'm not pregnant or anything, just really hungry!

You all know the feeling: Promising yourself that after just one more hot fudge sundae—which would make it an even ten for the night—you're going to put away the junk food forever and start eating right. Tomorrow, you tell yourself, that's when you're going to get off your fat butt and do something about your fat butt. But you want to know the truth? Ninety-eight percent of all diets don't work. So why bother? You're just putting yourself through hell so you can gain all the weight back and end up even fatter than when you started.

Name a diet, I've tried it. I've tried everything from group meetings to individual therapy, from liquid dinners to solid cardboard food, from Overeaters Anonymous to Fat Slobs United, from books and videos to powders and creams. I've tried Jenny Haag, Weight

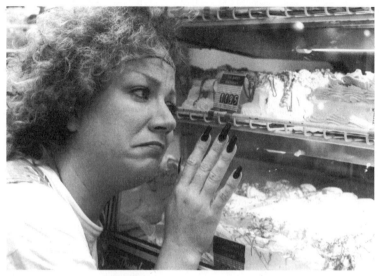

Remember the old days? Just you, me, and a bevnap.

Watchers, NutriSystem, and Jiffy Lube. I've also gone through all the same irrational, desperate, crazy schemes that all fat people dream up to make themselves thin, like tying myself to 18-wheelers when I go jogging or converting all my calories to Celsius. I've even traveled to Lourdes.

Once I tried nailing shut all the kitchen cabinets and throwing away the hammer. That night, I woke up at 2:00 A.M. and all I could think about was food. Guess what I did? I ate through the cabinet like a beaver. Using nothing but my two front teeth, I gnawed through three full inches of Formica and pressure-treated fiberboard. That night I discovered just how good drywall, grout, and penny nails could taste. The beautiful thing was, all those building supplies didn't just

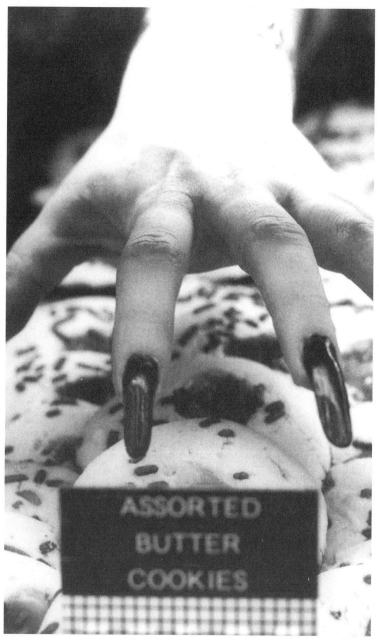

Ah, my three favorite things: assorted, butter, and cookies.

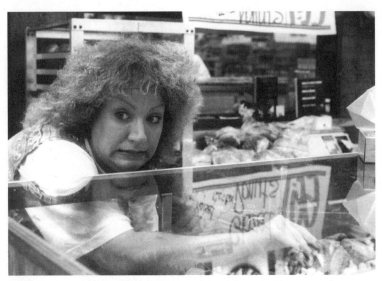

The secret to shopping is never looking guilty...

TASTE good, they were good <u>for</u> me, too! Low in fat, high in protein and carbohydrates. Believe me, you don't know what a high-fiber diet is until you've tried wood shavings! When I got to the food, I ate it all, too.

But trust me, none of these ridiculous diet schemes work. They're just modern medicine shows, nothing but cheap gimmicks that desperate people like you and me are all too happy to buy into. So save your precious time, money, energy, and calories. But don't worry, at the end of this chapter, I will tell you about the best way I ever found to lose weight.

Remember, 98 percent of all diets don't work. You want to know why? Read on.

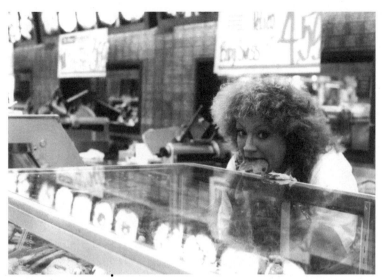

... and acting natural.

GETTING STARTED

It seems as though whenever I want to start a diet (Did I say that?) or a work-out program, the first thing I have to do is fill out some stupid questionnaire that gives my "supervisor" more information about me than anyone has a right to know. After all, when you go to a priest and confess to murder, all he wants to know is how long it's been since your last confession.

Not only are these questionnaires humiliating, embarrassing, and a complete violation of privacy, but I also can't see the point in them. Does anyone really need all of this information, and if they do, shouldn't they at least read me my Miranda rights first? I think the interrogations were easier when the Gestapo showed up at your door.

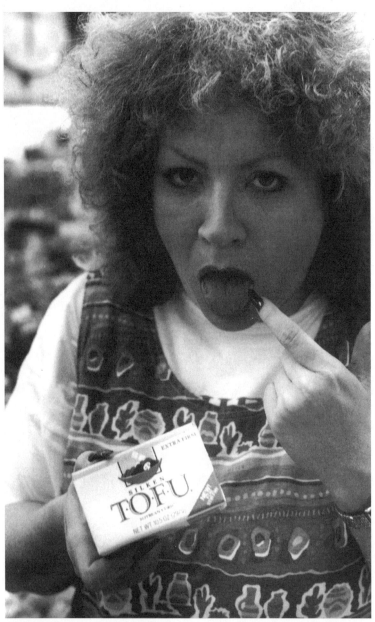

Tofu? Wasn't he David Carradine's character on that TV show?

While I am completely opposed to filling out these awful things, in the interest of full disclosure, I want to show the sample questionnaire I had to fill out at one diet place. (The next time you try a diet, feel free to substitute my answers for your own.)

Name: Beth Donahue
Age: 32
Occupation: Stand-up comedian
Height: 5'7" (I don't like where this is headed.)
Weight: Who wants to know? (See, I told you!)
What was your first experience with exercise?: When I was a little girl, in the days before the remote control was invented, my dad would scream at the top of his lungs and tell me to come downstairs and change the channel for him. That way, he could watch sports all weekend without having to get out of his chair. (Guess who I take after?)
How often do you exercise?: Three weeks before a date, a high school reunion, or whenever I see myself on television. I hate that.
How do you feel after a workout?: Resentful, bitter, weak, angry, fat, hopeless, ugly, suicidal, and hungry.
When you are working out, what images do you visualize for inspiration?: Shelley Winters, Larry "Bud" Melman, and Orson Welles. All naked.
What have you accomplished through sports?:

Exercise has helped me develop spider veins, a passionate hatred of Lycra, and a bad attitude. I have also learned that the Thighmaster can be used to crack walnuts.

Now that we have those gruesome details out of the way, let's talk about why diets don't work.

THE DIET INDUSTRY

What really kills me are the diets I see advertised in magazines, on television, and on the back of tubes of cookie dough. Somehow I don't get the feeling that the road to salvation begins with a magazine that features a skinny supermodel on the cover and articles about how to keep a man happy. If you want to keep the men I

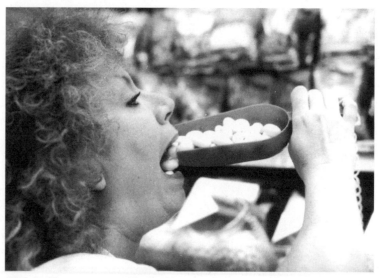

Take all you want. Eat all you take.

know happy, you don't have to read an article in a magazine, just give him a picture (or better yet, a video) of the supermodel on the cover.

I'm not sure where that leaves the rest of us, those who have tried just about every diet under the sun, know they don't work, and are still stupid enough to think that the fantastic new doctor-approved, previously-undiscovered-but-guaranteed-to-work-or-we'll-give-you-all-your-money-back diet (advertised next to the article about finding your G-spot—I say, if you need directions, ask at a gas station) is going to do the trick. We all know the diet is just some get-rich-quick scheme dreamt up by some fool who didn't have the time, energy, or brains to enroll in that art school you read about

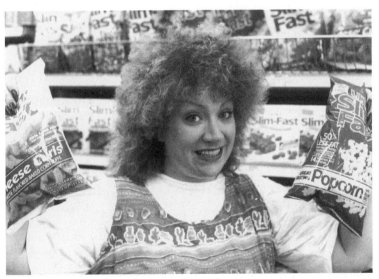

One for Zsa Zsa, one for Eva!

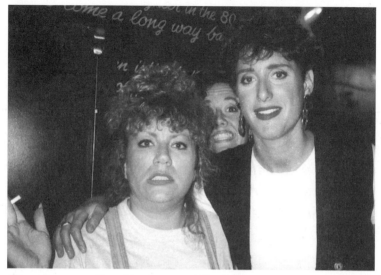

The picture of health (me and Judy Gold).

on matchbook covers. Let's face it, you don't need a degree in nutrition to take out a magazine advertisement and open up a post office box.

Still, we go along with it. We send in a check or money order made out to some fictitious doctor or make-believe Swedish clinic that has just discovered the cure for cellulite and is going to win a Nobel prize for their efforts. Then we're surprised when the diet doesn't work—and neither does the money-back guarantee.

One of my favorite diet ads is headlined, "When My Skinny Doctor Laughed at Me, I Actually Threw My Dress at Him." I like to call it, "When My Skinny Doctor Threw His Dress at Me, I Actually Laughed at Him." It's one of those really clever ads written up to

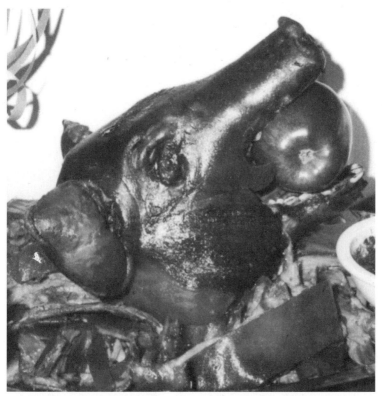

My future wedding cake... no wait, it's my ex-boyfriend.

<u>look</u> like a magazine article, but then they print the word ADVERTISEMENT at the top of the page so that you, dear reader, understand that this is <u>not</u> an actual article. Presumably they perform this noble public service to keep you from falling under the mistaken impression that it actually is one of those other reputable articles in the magazine that tell you how to use your breasts to build your career. Isn't it nice of the editors to tell us that this is an "ADVERTISEMENT"? (When the last paragraph of the article tells you to send

money to an address with which you're not familiar, it's so easy to mistake it for journalism, isn't it?)

Like so many other "can't-miss" diet plans, this one begins with a personal testimonial, which goes something like this:

"Hello, my name is Beth Donahue, and you don't know me from Adam. (Adam Rich, that is, the kid from "Eight is Enough," just about the only celebrity who doesn't have some kind of diet or exercise tape out there on the market these days.) But I'm not a celebrity, I'm a real person. (Truth be known, I'd rather be a celebrity, since the parties are a lot more fun, but right now I'm stuck with being a real person.) I live near Dallas, Texas, so you know I'm a real person—because no celebrity in his or her right mind would live here.

"I used to be fat. REALLY fat. So fat, in fact, that when I wanted to wear perfume, I had to buy it by the gallon and put it on with a turkey baster.

"Until two years ago, I was the fat lady everyone wanted to stand next to. (When you're really fat, other women want to stand near you because the trick to looking thin when you're heavy is to stand next to someone who is fatter than you are.) In the beginning, I thought this was a great idea—with so many women wanting to stand near me, I made lots of new friends, especially when I was in the nutrition section of the bookstore or the diet-food aisle at the grocery.

"But it got to the point where I had close to 419 people who insisted on standing by me all the time.

(I know that number seems large, but it's only a rough estimate. Let's just say you needed to know advanced calculus to keep track of all of them.) At first, it wasn't so much of a problem. Since I couldn't get to the refrigerator, I lost nearly 120 pounds! And since the other women surrounding me COULD get to the fridge, they all ballooned up to around 300 pounds. Eventually, this got to be a drag; being surrounded by a marching-band-size crowd of fat women makes it sort of hard to get a date. Plus there was a pretty good chance that in a few more days, we were actually going to begin orbiting the sun."

You know the story. The diet ad goes on and on and on with the personal testimonials. By the time you've read to the end, you're actually convinced: Yes! This is it! This is the one for me! The diet that's really going to work and put me out of my misery!!!

Well, I'm here to tell you not to believe it. It's not going to work, and you and I both know why: Any diet that's advertised in a magazine isn't worth the paper your hot check is written on. It's a waste of time, money, and calories. If you don't believe, take a look at the fine print.

First of all, most of these diets tell you right off the bat how much fun they're going to be because . . . you guessed it! YOU CAN EAT AS MUCH AS YOU WANT!!! If you're like me, you're already doing that and you already know what the results are.

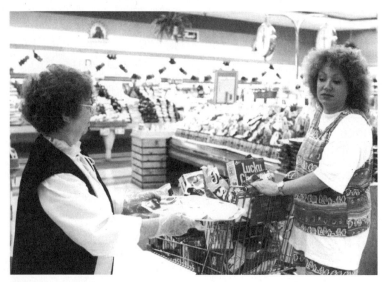

Woman meets woman…

Those all-you-can-eat diets always tell you the same lie right up front. It goes something like this, "The program worked because it was so simple. I ate ALL THE TIME! I could eat twelve times a day, so I never felt hungry. If I felt like a snack, I had one. I had a snack before breakfast, lunch, and dinner. I even had a snack before I had a snack. I ate as much as I wanted to, and I STILL lost weight!"

Stop right there, folks. I've checked all of these diets out, and I'm gonna tell you how they do it. Yes, it's true that you can eat as much as you want, but what they don't tell you is <u>what</u> you "get to" eat. For example, on one diet that's currently big in California, you can "eat as much as you want," but you can choose items only from the following list:

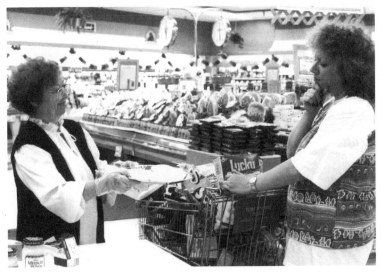

Woman makes peace offering.

   1. dillweed
   2. chickpeas
   3. tartar sauce
   4. mucous
   5. Tonka Toys
   6. wood chips
   7. balsa beams
   8. peanuts (the Styrofoam ones used in packing crates)
   9. dandelions
 10. broken watches

Sound like fun? I don't think so.

Next, they tell you why you've never heard about this diet before. It's never because the diet doesn't work or because it's only available to doctors—or because it's

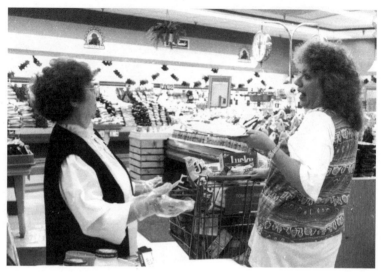

Shocked woman accepts offer…

so dangerous that even Oprah wouldn't try it. No! No! No! You just haven't heard of the diet before because "IT'S THE BEST-KEPT SECRET IN AMERICA!!" Thank God! It's good to know that the CIA has been keeping busy since the Berlin Wall came down. It's one thing to let the Soviets learn our state secrets or the North Koreans develop a nuclear bomb, but as long as we can keep this secret dietary information from falling into enemy hands, we can make sure the world remains safe for democracy.

Finally, the diet ad will tell you all the other reasons to send in your $350. (That's six easy monthly installments and your first-born child, an easy one-time-only installment.) The diet people also will tell you all about

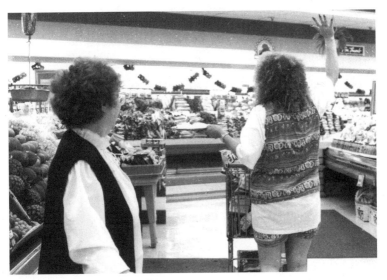

Women become friends.

the diet's "other great benefits." These usually include at least one of the following:

1. THIS DIET DOES NOT USE AMPHETAMINES.

Well, damn it, then I'm out. That's usually the main reason I want to go on a diet in the first place.

2. THIS DIET DOES <u>NOT</u> INVOLVE STRENUOUS EXERCISE PROGRAMS.

I have to admit, I fall for this one every time. It sounds too great to be true, yet I'm almost dumb enough to believe it. Let's face it, if you're too lazy to move your big butt off the Barcolounger, you're probably not going to drop much tonnage.

3. ON THIS DIET, YOU DO NOT COUNT CALORIES.

They supply a little Asian boy who follows you around with an abacus and does the counting for you.

4. YOU CAN DINE OUT.

Sure you can, as long as you can find a restaurant that serves water and Melba toast. (Most do.)

5. ONCE YOU LOSE THE WEIGHT, YOU'LL KEEP IT OFF! WE GUARANTEE IT!

You know why they guarantee it? Because the diet is so unbelievably dangerous that if you actually stick to it, it will kill you. That's right, you'll be so thin, you'll be able to wear anything you want . . . to your own funeral. And once you've moved on to the great All-You-Can-Eat dessert bar in the sky, you won't be able to sue the damn company that suckered you into the stupid diet in the first place. Dead people can't sue, that's how these guys make their money.

Remember, when it comes to diets ads, the bottom line is: if it sounds too good to be true, it is. There's no such thing as a free lunch—especially when you're fat. I know, because I've been looking for one for the last 15 years. So if you want to be a mindless idiot and fall for yet another insane diet that will break your bank account, go ahead and send in your life's savings. As for me, I'm sick of falling hook, line, and sinker for this tired old copywriter bait. I'd rather save my money and spend it on something that's really important to me—like chili dogs, ice cream sundaes, and candy bars.

EATING DISORDERS

An area not traditionally known for its rich vein of humor is eating disorders. Comedians have always made their living telling fat jokes, not skinny jokes (other than during times of famine, that is). If most people thought there was anything funny about anorexia and bulimia, Roseanne would have killed herself and Olive Oyl would have the highest-rated sitcom on TV. Eating disorders are nothing more than the product of society's ridiculous expectations for women and their bodies. Between movies, television, and magazine covers, not to mention an entire industry built around Cindy Crawford, you can't swing a stale cupcake without hitting the image of a super-thin, super-sexy supermodel who only got to be so thin because her diet consists solely of speed and vodka. (Some things you learn in high school can be used later in life; now, if someone would just find a practical use for calculus). As for the super-thin, super-sexy actress, trust me, she got her body through plastic surgery.

At this point it's a cliché to complain about how the media gives women negative images of their own bodies, and I certainly don't want to blame anyone else for they way I look. But let's face it, if I didn't feel like I had to compete with all those bikini-clad bimbos in beer commercials, I wouldn't place so many unrealistic expectations on my own body. I don't know about you, but for me, these expectations range from wanting to

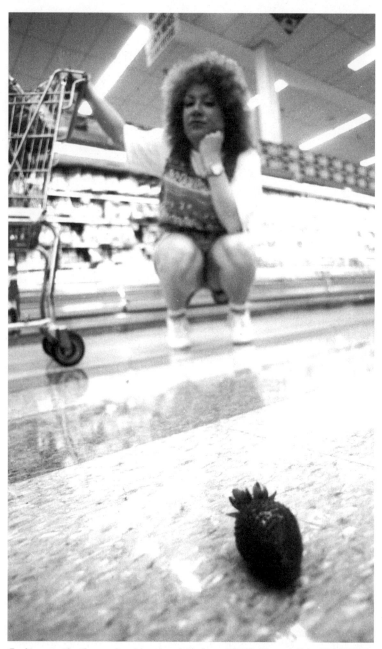

Is it worth the calories to pick it up? Hell no! It's FRUIT!

look good in a bathing suit and being able to wear a skin-tight miniskirt to getting out of bed in the morning without using a hydraulic lift.

I've always found that as with most other things in life, blaming my parents or my boyfriend always makes me feel better, at least in the short run. But whether or not you choose to blame your weight problems on someone else, there's no denying that anorexia and bulimia are serious problems that shouldn't be taken lightly. (But then again, I'm a comedian, so what the hell.)

I can't say that I don't understand anorexia, because Lord knows, I too have looked in the mirror and seen a fabulous body trapped under layer upon layer of fat that shouldn't be there. Of course, what I'm seeing is an illusion brought on by the light-headedness that comes from eating one lone Cheerio for breakfast. For me, the delusion is that I'm only 80 pounds overweight instead of 100. This fantasy is brought on by the sugar high that comes after I eat a whole box of Cap'N Crunch as a snack before I head out for the All-You-Can-Eat breakfast bar at Shoney's.

But after a delusional session in front of the mirror, I can't say I really get the whole concept of anorexia. I don't want to sound unsympathetic. Believe me, I am sympathetic. I really am. An eating disorder is an eating disorder, and I know anorexia is a serious problem. But let me just say that when you weigh 230 pounds and you're tired of going to the drive-through car wash every time you need a shower, anorexia is a problem you sometimes wish you had. I know such a confession may sound gruesome, but it's true. There have been times when I was so desperate to lose weight that I would seek out people with anorexia and kiss them full on the mouth, just so that I could catch it. Sounds sick, I know, but that's pretty much all you need to know about what dieting can do to a person. (This was before we knew how dangerous anorexia is, to say nothing of the fact that people can die from it. But then again, I haven't seen any of my ribs in five years. I have no idea what color my toenails are, and I can pretty much forget about buying shoes with laces. That doesn't sound a whole lot safer, does it?)

As for bulimia, well, I've tried vomiting, but then again, who hasn't? Pretty much every woman I know has stuck her fingers down her throat at some point in her life, although most of them do it just because Michael Bolton is on the radio. One bulimic friend took a trip to Mexico and drank tap water every chance she got, just hoping she would catch some horrible tropical disease that would give her diarrhea. Now that's sick.

But the bottom line with barfing is that I really don't understand the point of it all. When I put three large orders of McDonald's French fries in my belly, I want to keep them there. I don't want them coming back up! I want them to enjoy their new happy home in my gut. And if they get lonely, I'll gladly send down a Big Mac or two to keep them company. So I'm glad to say, and grateful for the fact, that the dietus vomitorium never worked for me.

I must admit, however, that back in high school, when I was the life of the party, I often practiced the "throwing up" diet unintentionally. So if, after consulting with your doctor and your plumber (since you will be using the toilet quite frequently), you decide you must throw up and can't, give this tried and true technique a shot:

1. Eat two-three bean burritos without pausing for air.
2. Do shots of Seagrams 7 in multiples of seven.

That should pretty much do the trick.

These days, of course, bulimia doesn't just mean throwing up. It also means purging your body using laxatives. I find this method particularly ridiculous, because who wants to spend all day on the can? Plus, in a world where so many people spend so much money on Metamucil, Ex-Lax, Correctol, prune juice, high-fiber cereals, and just about anything short of garden mulch, it just doesn't seem right to spend so much time in the bathroom when so many others are spending so much time and energy just trying to get there.

If you insist on going this route, you can always fall back on my personal favorite diet, pancake batter and prune juice—the Flap 'n' Crap Diet. All you need to do is buy both and consume as much as possible of each. As long as the quantities are roughly equal, they pretty much cancel each other out.

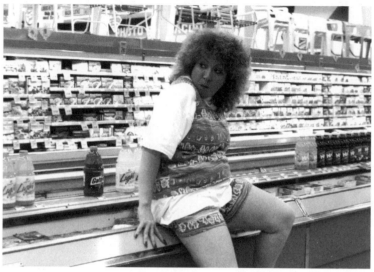

Slowly, I turn…

OTHER DIETS

Name a diet, and I've tried it. Let's go down the list, shall we?

Jenny Haag

My God in heaven, if you're thinking about joining Jenny Haag, I think you might as well just take all your money and flush it right down the toilet, because the bottom line is that's where it's going to end up anyway. It's a whole lot quicker, a whole lot easier, and a whole lot more realistic this way, plus there's always the chance that when those greenbacks clog up your toilet, the plumber who comes out to fix it will be that hunky dreamboat you've been waiting for. (You and I both know that every plumber in the world is really a fat,

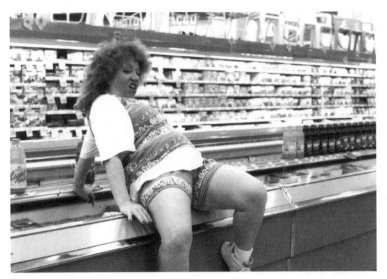

Step by step. Inch by inch…

drunken slob who can't read and walks around with his
pants halfway down his butt. But if you believe the fantasy that Jenny Haag will work for you, you'll believe
just about anything.)

Now, to their credit, the people at Jenny Haag have
their hearts in the right place. It's just their brains I'm
worried about. These good folks want to "re-train" your
eating habits. While this may sound like a good idea,
trust me, it doesn't work. That's the first problem. The
second problem is that "re-training" your eating habits
is the most banal, humiliating thing I have ever been
through.

I remember sitting in one of my "classes" at Jenny
Haag with my "counselor," a Heather Locklear clone
who knew what it was like to be overweight because

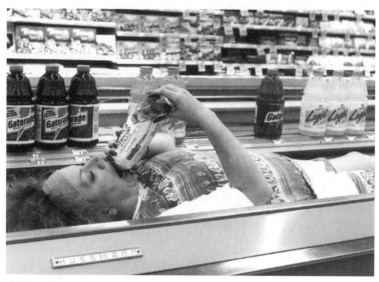

Dinner!

she herself once had to haul around eight extra pounds! I know every detail about this tragic period in her life because she told us about it with tears in her eyes. Somehow, she managed to turn this isolated incident of personal trauma into a five-part miniseries that covered the bulk of our first week together. The whole time I was there, all I could think was "Eight pounds??!!" Each one of my boobs weighs eight pounds!

The really annoying thing is the way these counselors talk to you—like you're seven years old and you can't control your own body and its urges. (Which, of course, you can't. If you could, you wouldn't be there in the first place, but that's not my point). I remember one class where the topic was, "WHAT TO DO WHEN

YOU'RE EATING OUT." My counselor actually said, "Okay, the dessert cart is coming around. Everyone at the table is looking at you. How do you say no??!!"

She seemed to think that when I go to a restaurant with friends, they sit around chanting, "Eat it! Eat it! Eat it! C'mon, all your friends are doing it!" What kind of people did she think I hang around with? I KNOW the difference between dinner at a restaurant and a high school pep rally. It's not like my friends and I build a bonfire whenever we go out to eat—unless I'm in the mood for barbecue.

And had my counselor seen some special X-rays of me with no spine? I can say "no" to some things. You know, when they're important. Like heroin, dental surgery, and sixth helpings. Plus, if I really felt like I had to make an excuse for turning down dessert, I would just say, "No thanks, the 68-ounce porterhouse steak was plenty." (Not that I would ever turn down the dessert cart.)

And the ads for Jenny Haag are incredible: "Join this week for free!" they scream, as if it's really not going to cost you one red cent to drop the extra body you're carrying around. Just be sure to bring in a bond to cash in so you can afford the food.

As expensive as it is, the food at Jenny Haag (to their credit) is not all bad. The pancakes are to die for. They might taste good, but let's face it, you need to eat 48 of them just to dent your hunger. I've seen bigger portions in doll houses. Besides, the whole time I was on their food, all I could think was, "God, I can't wait for this crap to end so I can eat REAL food again!" And that, in the end, is the real problem with Jenny Haag and everyone else like her. NO ONE CAN RE-TRAIN YOU TO EAT!

Weight Watchers

Same story here, folks. I'm sorry, but counting calories just isn't for me. I never liked math to begin with and I know that as soon as I start counting anything, that tells me just one thing: I have to stop counting sometime, which means I'm never going to be able to eat as much as I want to on this diet.

The other problem with Weight Watchers and all the other franchises is that I'm never going to be able to trust <u>any</u> diet center that's located in a strip mall. I'm sorry, but I go to the mall to shop, not to lose weight. And isn't it just a little ridiculous to put the weight-loss clinic in the middle of the strip center next to This Can't Be Yogurt?

The Scarsdale Diet

Great idea, but again, calorie counting. They say the nice thing about this diet is that when you're on it, you can eat all the fruit you want. You already know how I feel about that! Big deal! If nature makes it and it's good for you, then I don't want anything to do with it. As far as I'm concerned, fruit is not food. It's fruit. It's empty. It's tasteless, and every time I eat it I'm <u>starving</u> all day.

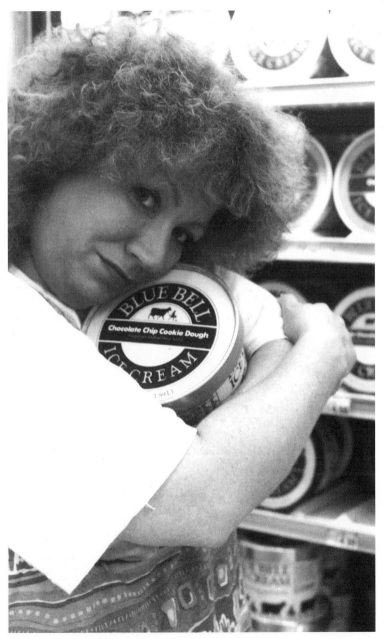

Mommy misses you, too.

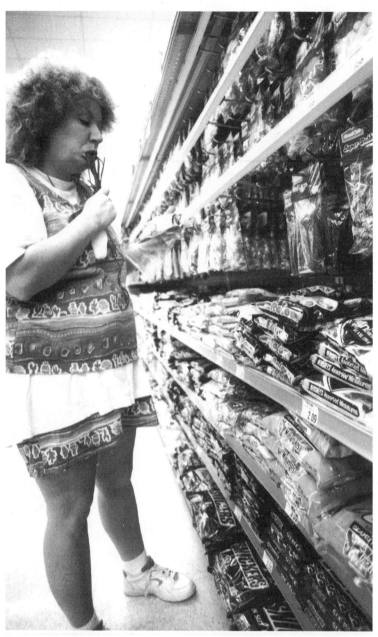

Life truly is a buffet.

Besides, all you need to know about the Scarsdale Diet is what happened to the guy who invented it. You remember Dr. Herman Tarnower, don't you? He's the one who was allegedly assassinated by Jean Harris, the former headmistress at that tony girls boarding school. Let's face it, this is a story we can all relate to. But at the same time, when a diet kills a doctor, it kind of makes you wonder what it will do to the patients.

Overeaters Anonymous

I tried Overeaters Anonymous. Once. At the beginning of the meeting, everyone was crying and commiserating. Within fifteen minutes, we were all on a bus to The Sizzler. I don't remember how we got from point A to point B, but I figured I better not go back.

Liquid Diets

Here's what I think about Slim Fast and all its bastard cousins: A shake for breakfast, a shake for lunch, a shake as a snack, a shake for dinner, a shake before you go to bed at night, and a puke fest at midnight. Get up in the morning, your butt is still shaking.

Cremes, Gels, and Jellies

They don't remove cellulite and they don't make you thinner. Period. End of story. If you really want a topical application that will make your skin disappear, you're better off contracting that new flesh-eating strep bacteria. It's the only thing that works.

Personal Trainers, Dietitians, and Nutritionists

Personally, I think Oprah is the coolest. I could lose 100 pounds too if I had a team of 55 doctors, chefs, dietitians, psychologists, and game wardens following me around 24 hours a day. The only problem with this method is that if I could afford to pay someone to <u>make</u> the crap for me, then I might consider eating it. But I don't have the cash, and to make matters worse, I also don't like most of the food these people make you eat. Which brings me to . . .

Other Gimmicks

I absolutely hate any person or program that tells you to "Write down everything you eat." You should hate them too. They tell you that when you actually see all your food on paper you will be horrified by what you have written down (the same feeling Ivana Trump must have each time she finishes a novel). First of all, I can't eat and write at the same time, and when it comes down to choosing one of them, I think you know which one I'm going to go with.

When I do take a time-out from stuffing my face, the idea of sitting there trying to remember everything I've just eaten can be difficult. And once I do pause, it's so easy for something small—a turkey or a wedding cake—to slip my mind. I can't tell you how many times that has happened.

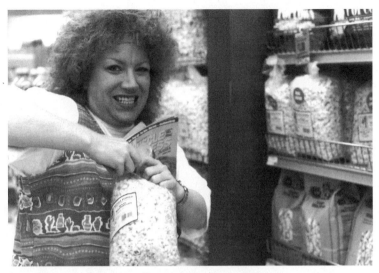

I need to work out so I can open my snacks.

TWO DIETS THAT <u>DO</u> WORK

The Spider Diet

This is by far the safest, most effective diet I have ever tried. The only problem is, it's very difficult to duplicate.

Way back in 1982, I woke up one morning with a huge bite on my backside. I couldn't figure out how I ended up with a giant bite on my butt, but since Ted Bundy was in jail, I figured that I had either gotten way too drunk the night before or I had been attacked by some kind of insect. I went to the doctor and found out that it was indeed a spider bite.

The doctor told me that it would get a lot bigger (I think he was talking about the bite, not my butt) and

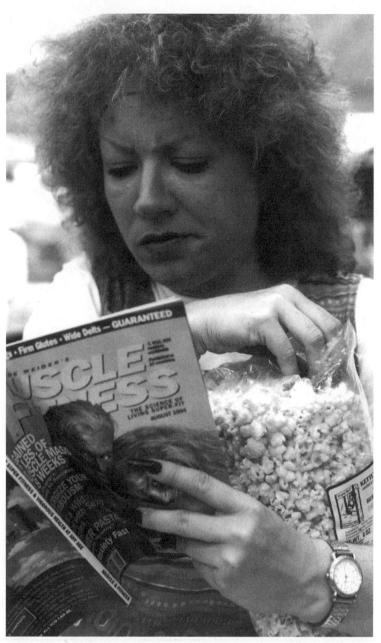

What's wrong with this picture?

that it would itch like nobody's business. In case you're wondering, there is no way to scratch your butt in public without constantly backing into things, so you can guess how ridiculous I looked.

The spider bite got bigger and itchier for THREE FULL MONTHS. It turned out to be the most hideous, annoying thing I have ever suffered through in my life—yes, including relationships. But there was one saving grace, a blessed and divine side effect that I had not counted on: For these three months, I could not put one bite of food in my mouth without wanting to puke. Believe me, I tried, but nothing tasted good: not McDonald's French fries, not wedding cake, not cookie dough. You name it, I couldn't eat it.

For some reason, the good Lord had decided in His infinite wisdom to send me a natural appetite suppressant, via divine intervention! All of a sudden, I was wearing a size 7, the same size as the dress I wore for my first communion. My mother even said the words we all dream of hearing: "You're too thin. You look sick." I was in heaven.

Of course, it did not last. Just as the itch went away, my appetite came back and so did the weight. I've been looking for that spider ever since. I know if I could just find that damn thing, breed it, and sell its offspring in jars, I would be a millionaire. (I still go to the deepest, darkest of wooded areas and roll around naked for hours, but I haven't gotten lucky—with the spider or anyone else.)

The Mafia Diet

In 1986 I was at my absolute thinnest. Unfortunately, the secret of my success wasn't a pleasant one. My body was ravaged with drugs and alcohol, which is one easy, but definitely not recommended, way to stay thin.

To make matters worse—and me thinner—I was living with a guy who killed people for a living. Believe me, sharing a bed with a murderer is the best way I've ever found to keep the pounds off. As his body count kept going up, I was having a hard time keeping food down. I literally vomited with fear nearly every day of my life. Believe me, there's nothing like waking up in the middle of the night with a shotgun pointed at you to make those hunger pains vanish. The whole thing made the ending of *Goodfellas* look like an episode of "Leave it to Beaver." Eventually I realized I had to get out of that relationship, and luckily I had the courage to do so.

Of course, now I'd like to get back to being that shell of a person, but without costing so many people their lives (myself included.) Then again, one or two folks wouldn't be so bad—especially if they were weight-loss counselors at Jenny Haag—but mass murder and mayhem I can do without. The lesson here is that if you really want to lose a lot of weight fast, move in with a contract killer. I don't necessarily recommend it, but since John Gotti is looking for work, it just might do the trick!

The nice thing about this technique is that while it may jeopardize your life (every diet plan has some kind of unwanted side effect), you will learn a lot of interesting information that's hard to pick up anywhere else. Sure, it's a little dangerous, but let's see how it stacks up against other weight-loss plans.

Say you go to a Pritikin weight-loss center. All they're going to teach you is how to count calories, eat smarter, and maybe exercise a little bit everyday. A week at one of these grown-up fat camps is going to cost you upwards of $300,000, with .3 percent of that covered by health insurance, and you're not really going to learn anything you didn't know before, except to trade "how-to-cheat" secrets with other campers! Plus, if you really want to stay thin their way, you're going to spend most of your life savings buying their food for the next 20 years. You'll be thin and—maybe—happy, but your kids

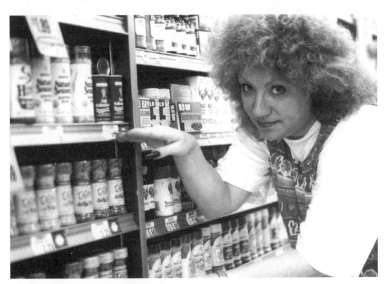

Mrs. Dash, Mrs. Butter, no salt, no flavor...

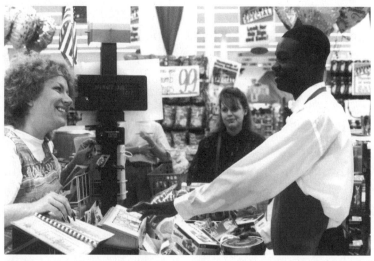

Paper, plastic, or do you just want to pull up a chair?

won't ever be able to go to college because you sank every penny you had into food that's about as much fun to eat as wet sawdust.

Now, if you move in with a guy who works for The Mob, you'll learn much more interesting stuff. For example, if you live with a Mafia-trained killer, you will learn:

1. How to swear in another language.
2. What "capice" means.
3. How to use a gun.
4. Where to buy sharkskin suits.
5. All about men's jewelry.
6. Handy places to hide a body.

The best thing about Mafia guys is that they really know how to cook. Pritikin will feed you a 4-ounce boneless, skinless, tasteless chicken breast cooked in turpentine with a side of two Brussels sprouts, and maybe for dessert they'll let you have a nice, tall, frosty glass of ice water. On the other hand, your Mafia boyfriend will put you on a steady diet of chicken, sausage, milk-fed veal, clams, pasta, mozzarella, Romano, parmesan, olive oil, rich cream sauces, and decadent tomato sauces (not to mention the delicious lead garnish). For dessert you'll enjoy a wide variety of exquisite Italian delights, all of them high in calories and pleasure. You'll eat like a mobster, and since you'll be a nervous, paranoid wreck all day, every day, there's absolutely no chance in hell that you'll ever be able to keep any of this wonderful food down. In other words, you'll never end up looking like Francis Ford Coppola.

The best thing about this diet plan is the price. None of this will cost you a cent. Of course, you might want to factor in what a good lawyer charges per hour, because if your man ever goes down, you are going to need someone to represent you. The government can and will charge you with aiding and abetting a known criminal, as well as your appetite! On the other hand, if you do go to prison, the food there is so horrible that you won't be able to do anything but lose weight. When you weigh your options, you win either way with this one.

Think about it. It really worked for me!

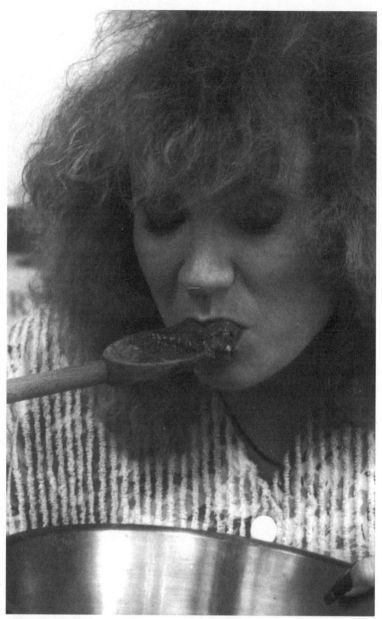

Double bubble toil and trouble...chocolate's done...and so's my hair!!

SIX

101 Creative Recipes for Cardboard

If I liked eating natural fiber, I would have eaten my roof by now.

DIET FOOD

This one's easy—stay away from diet food! It tastes like cardboard, the portions are tiny, and it's not as "low-cal" as they say it is. Basically, the diet industry looks at their pre-packaged food the way restaurants look at alcohol: it's where they make all their money. After they sign you up for next to nothing, they gouge you to death on this stuff. It's the equivalent of eating playing cards and it's just not worth it.

I love those food-garnishing kits that let you make all your food into animals. I like to make the San Diego Zoo. And making curly fries? As if I really need to make French fries more attractive in order to find them appetizing!

DIET RECIPES

Let me say right from the start that the only "special recipe" that I'm interested in is the Colonel's.

The problem with food that's "good for you" is that it's not good for your taste buds. Living off this stuff is not life as we know it. Besides, if I'm going to go to the trouble of cooking, I'm not going to prepare eggplant baguettes. I'm going to make Fifteen-Alarm Chili—and I'm going to put enough sour cream and cheese on it to make a dairy farmer blush.

My diet doctor insisted that I buy a book called *Eat More, Weigh Less,* because he said it had tons of "wonderful recipes" in it. To begin with, any recipe always "serves 6-10"—like I know ten people who really want to eat this crap! I think you and I both know what's going to happen if I cook enough food to serve that many people. That's right, it ends up serving one person—me (who didn't like the junk in the first place).

To make matters worse, I usually haven't heard of 98 percent of the ingredients in these recipes. You have to go to the sorcerer's shop to get half of them, and do you have any idea how expensive newts and toads are these days? Here's a list of some of the ingredients in these recipes in this book, *Eat More, Weigh Less.* Have you ever heard of any of them?

1. Fennel (Is this animal, vegetable, or mineral?)
2. Leeks (Huh?)
3. Dried kombu seaweed (What?)
4. Chervil (Even my grocer hasn't heard of this one.)
5. Chiffoneded fresh basil (Sounds like an all-girl band from the sixties.)
6. Fenugreek (Gezundheit!)
7. Turmeric (Isn't this what the plane taxis in on?)
8. Avosh, a large Armenian cracker bread disk (Will it fit in my CD player?)
9. Cardamom (A Balkan Mother's Day card?)
10. English cucumber
11. Hungarian paprika (might get in a fight with the English cucumber.)
12. Mirin (Even Martha Stewart never used this one.)
13. Grated lemon zest (Is this a new kind of soap?)
14. Fava beans
15. Yukon potatoes
16. Mung beans (No comment!)

Here's a list of the ingredients I have in my apartment. See if you can find any correlation between this one and the one above.

1. Butter
2. Lard
3. Crisco
4. Semi-sweet chocolate chips (Will do in a pinch for late-night binges.)

5. Baking soda
6. I Can't Believe It's Not Butter
7. This Can't Be Butter
8. I Wish It Were Butter
9. Sure Looks Like Butter
10. It's Not Really Salt
11. I Can't Believe It's Not Salt
12. I Can't Believe It's Not Lard
13. Cayenne Pepper
14. Original Mrs. Dash
15. Every other Mrs. Dash ever invented
16. I Can't Believe It's Not Mrs. Dash
17. Mr. Dash
18. Mr. Dash's Secretary
19. Mr. Dash's Illegitimate Son
20. Mr. Dash's Divorce Lawyer
21. Mr. Dash Meets Mrs. Butterworth

That's what I call a spice rack, and if a recipe calls for something I don't have in the house, then I'm just not going to bother with making it.

If you think the ingredients are ridiculous, you should see the recipes themselves. To begin with, they're incredibly violent: almost all the ingredients have to be "smashed," "beaten," "finely chopped," or "vivisected." Who's doing the cooking here, Clint Eastwood? But the worst part about this cookbook is that everything in it—just like all low-cal recipes—is incredibly time consuming and difficult, to say nothing of impractical. Here's what I'm talking about:

• Vegetables have to be roasted in the oven for an hour and stirred occasionally. How do I stir something that's in the oven? I'm not short enough to fit in there.

• You're supposed to let the vegetables "sweat." How? Do I put them in front of the TV and put Richard Simmons's *Sweatin' to the Veggies* tape in the VCR?

• Yogurt cheese, once made, should be stored for up to one week. I will have starved to death by then. But at least the recipe is so gross that I won't be tempted to eat it while I'm cooking.)

• They make a big deal about presentation. What fat person cares about presentation, much less cleansing her palate? Two gallons of root beer usually does the trick.

• Sauces can be stored in "cool, dark places" for up to three months. Behind my toilet would be a good place, but can I eat ANY of this stuff right away?

• The eggplant baguette is recommended for a tailgate party. Have you ever heard of anything so pretentious? "I know we usually have hot dogs, but does anybody want an eggplant baguette?"

• Split peas "take on a whole new dimension." What dimension did they used to be in? The Fifth?

• One sandwich recipe reminds you to "cover with a second slice of bread and cut in half." Thank God, I usually forget that part!

• Vegetarian chili is made from 23 different ingredients. There are more spare parts in the space shuttle. Just open up a can of Hormel.

Let's face it, these life-saving, low-cal recipes are just too much work for anyone who has even a part-time job. I don't know who they think has enough time to do all this work, much less has the interest to do it. And by the time I get all these ingredients shipped in from England, Japan, and the Yukon, I'll pretty much have starved to death. They should have just called this book, *Wait More, Eat Less.*

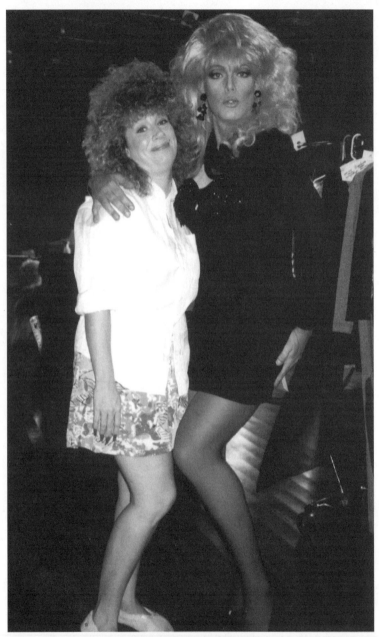

One of us has been surgically altered.

SEVEN

Never Consult a Physician

The diet pills that used to work are illegal. Today, the ones that are legal, don't.

The seeds of my addiction to diet pills were planted during high school. The old speed-and-vodka diet was my first experience with pill popping, and since then I've had plenty of experience. Trust me here, I know what I'm talking about.

I have taken a lot of diet pills, both legal and illegal, and so have you. Don't tell me that just because your doctor gave you a prescription that everything's on the up and up. You and I both know your doctor will give you any prescription you want if you whine and complain enough, so don't pretend that he's the one who's in control of the pharmacy. You are. And if you're not, I suggest you get yourself a new doctor.

I tried diet pills for the last time just this year and I wish I could tell you they still work. They don't. In all my years of taking diet pills, the only place I lost weight was in my mouth, since the stupid pills made me grind my teeth down to the nubs. I guess that would have been a good thing if having no teeth had kept my appetite down, but it didn't. All I ended up doing was chewing my food more. (Instead of once, I chewed it twice.)

On top of that, diet pills kept me up all night, so in the end I was still a fat slob, but one who was a whole lot grumpier before breakfast. A breakfast that, by the way, was still as big as it was before I started taking doctor-prescribed speed. So quit wasting your money. Those pills don't do a damn thing, which is just further

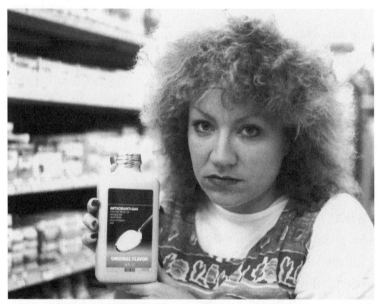

A food addict's best friend.

proof that medicine is still the most backward science known to man.

> I had a doctor who once spent 45 minutes telling me how to chew. I think it's obvious I've got that one down, Doc!

As far as I'm concerned, the only thing diet doctors are good for is drugs. Diet pills may not work, but anytime you can get a prescription for something, I definitely think it's worth the effort. If you go to a diet doctor, the bottom line is that he's going to tell you that you have to do two things if you want to lose weight:

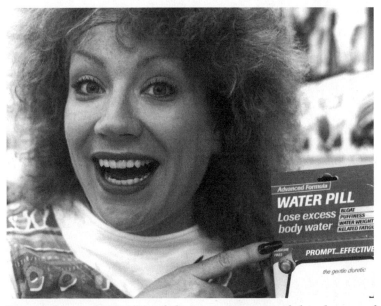

You only need 38,000 of these to get your eight glasses of water per day.

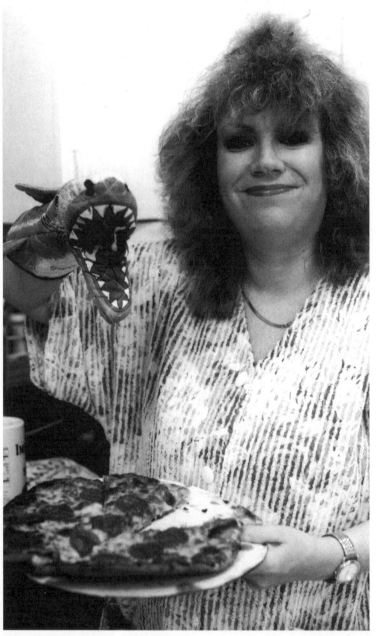

The puppet gets just one piece.

1. Change your eating habits
   and/or
2. Exercise.

I don't like either of these options. I think you already know how I feel about exercise, so we'll deal with the other scenario here.

CHANGING YOUR EATING HABITS

We all know the story of how Moses came down from the mountaintop with the Ten Commandments written on two stone tablets. If you've ever been to a diet doctor, you already know that most of them have a Moses complex—which is kind of like thinking you're Jesus, but the ending is a lot happier. Every diet doctor I've ever been to has given me a list of commandments that I absolutely, positively <u>must</u> follow if I'm ever going to get thin. Just like the Ten Commandments, they look really good on stone and it doesn't seem like they should be that hard to follow. And just like the Ten Commandments, they ARE hard to follow—not to mention the fact that they take all the fun out of life.

My diet doctor is just like all the others. I love the guy, but he told me losing weight would be easy, that all I had to do was change my eating habits. Then he gave me a list of six rules to follow. They went something like this:

The Six Commandments of Your New Eating Behavior

1. Place all food to be eaten on one plate.

2. Be seated at your designated place for eating or drinking.

3. Take three deep and relaxing breaths before eating.

4. Place your spoon or fork on your plate after each bite.

5. Chew your food until it has a liquid consistency.

6. Leave the table immediately after eating.

In the first place, I kind of like my eating habits the way they are, thank you very much. They may not be perfect, but at this point, the way I eat is second nature. Besides, if a habit works for me, I stick with it. I don't care whether it's smoking, chewing gum, or taking the trash out once a year (option: put a dumpster next to your couch). In the second place, if eating habits were that easy to change, we all would have done so already. The truth is, eating habits are just about impossible to change, so I suggest you do what I do—DON'T WORRY ABOUT IT! Besides, it's not like these commandments are written in stone or anything.

The one thing I DO like about this whole Ten Commandment analogy is that when it comes to dieting and commandments, I feel just like Moses: I've been wandering in the desert for about 30 years and I still don't have a clue where I'm going. In fact, the only difference between me and Moses is that they didn't have drive-through windows in his day to make life on the road easier. (Come to think of it, there is one other difference between me and Moses: if I ever came across a burning

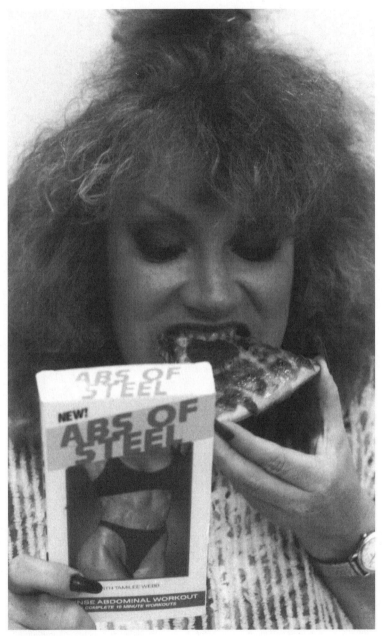

Abs of steel; jaws of life.

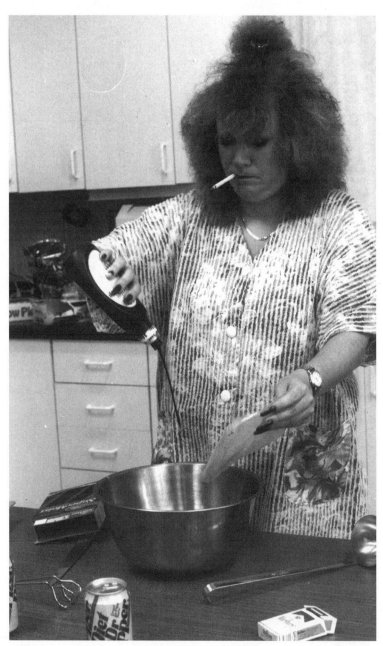

Glamour Shots, eat your heart out!

bush, I'd be sure to roast some marshmallows and make up a batch of s'mores before I started talking to God.)

I'm sure your diet doctor has given you some annoying list of commandments or lifestyle changes. And I'm sure that if you've tried them, you're just as frustrated as I am with the whole thing. But don't worry, I've got the solution for you. I've switched around the traditional commandments to make them a little more realistic and a lot easier to follow. So sit down, take a load off, and belly up to the dinner table. And remember, if at any point during the meal you are not enjoying your food, put some more butter on it!

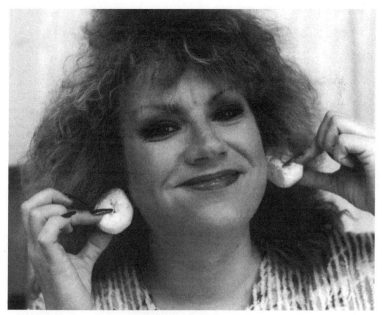

Earrings by Dunkin Donuts.

Beth's Ten Commandments

1. PLACE ALL FOOD TO BE EATEN ON ONE PLATTER—preferably one that is no smaller than a monster truck hubcap. Experts tell you that it is important that you be able to see the total amount of food you plan to eat before you take your first bite. This way, you can gauge how long you can eat before you blow an artery—and you can call ahead to make sure an ambulance is standing by. Also, avoid eating from:

    a. the back seat of your car

    b. between the cushions of your couch

    c. another person's mouth

    d. trash cans.

2. BE SEATED AT YOUR DESIGNATED PLACE OF EATING—which means you should always call ahead to make a reservation at Bennigan's, Chili's, TGI Friday's, or your mother's house.

3. THINK OF EATING AS A SEPARATE EXPERIENCE. In other words, don't confuse it with activities that you find unpleasant, such as cleaning your bathroom, changing diapers, or spending time with your children. (I used to have trouble following this commandment. For a long time, I confused going to the rodeo with being at one of those Chinese restaurants where they show you your food live before they cook it for you. I just thought the portions at the rodeo were larger.)

4. AVOID STANDING OR WALKING WHILE EATING. It's a real drag trying to carve a Thanksgiving turkey while you're on a hike with your friends.

5. DO NOT TAKE <u>ANY</u> DEEP BREATHS BEFORE EATING. If you do and you're like me, your food will disappear.

6. DO <u>NOT</u> PUT DOWN YOUR SPOON OR FORK AFTER EACH MOUTHFUL. I prefer eating with tongs. Diet doctors say that holding your eating utensil while chewing just encourages preparation for your next mouthful. Well, of course it does, but it's not like I need encouragement! The mere sight of the tongs leaving my mouth brings up all of my abandonment issues, and I feel sick until I feel the reassuring touch of steel on my lips once again.

7. TAKE MORE TIME EATING—AS MUCH AS POSSIBLE. I usually schedule a couple of hours for breakfast and like to make lunch last long enough to take me all the way into dinner.

8. CHEW YOUR FOOD ONCE. If you chew your food until it has a liquid consistency, then it's not really food anymore! If I'm not CHEWING, then I'm not EAT-ING! Doctors say that chewing allows a greater number of taste sensations to reach the hunger center in your brain. Great! But my hunger center is in my stomach!

9. LEAVE THE TABLE IMMEDIATELY AFTER EATING. This is a great idea, especially if you're at a really expensive restaurant and your Visa card is maxed out.

10. WHEN YOU FEEL HUNGRY, START ALL OVER AGAIN WITH NUMBER ONE! Enough said.

HEALTH ISSUES

Diabetes is one of the big health issues among people who are overweight. My dad has had it for years. He's just like me, he loves to eat. All he does is sit in the La-Z-Boy and eat ice cream, which I think is the prescription for diabetes.

One of the things about diabetes is that people with it often lose all sense of feeling in their hands and feet. My dad hasn't felt his hands or feet in ten years, so when he's driving, he never knows if his foot is on the gas or the brake. Last summer, he barbecued his hand. I had to tell him, "Dad, you're on fire again!"

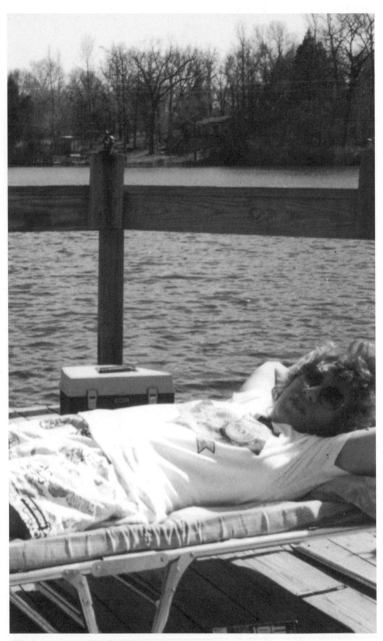

Wake me up before you go-go.

EIGHT

No One Looks Good in a Thong

If you don't have oxygen, you die.
—Susan Powter
If you don't have food, you starve.
—Beth Donahue

People often ask me if they should consult with a doctor before starting an exercise program. "You can do whatever you want," I tell them. "But if I were you, I wouldn't start an exercise program."

The bottom line with me and exercise is that we don't get along. Not because it's work (which I also don't like), but because I am lazy. Laziness is my natural state. As you know, the laws of physics, which govern the workings of the natural world, tell us that bodies at rest tend to stay at rest. I don't know about you, but I find it pretty hard to argue against the underlying forces of the universe.

The problem is this: Society has ruined laziness for us. Not too long ago, it used to be okay to stay in bed all day. Nobody cared if you did it, because they were doing it, too. But nowadays, if you lie in bed all day, people start whispering behind your back, "Oh, she must be depressed." I'm not depressed, I'm just tired!

People do the same thing with eating. Everyone always says, "Oh, she eats so much. She must be feeding her inner-child issues." Look, people, I'm just feeding my outer adult. I don't have any inner-child issues— I just love food! So get off my back.

One of the reasons I'm so lazy is that I love BED. Not sex, just bed. I love everything about the bed—sheets, pillows, blankets, dreams, rolling around—I just love it. So why can't I stay in it? If I'm a stand-up comic and I don't have to be at work until 8:00 P.M., who's to tell me I can't stay in bed? The bottom line is, I love lying down. Period. Anywhere most people stand, I lay down. In airports, the DMV, the lines at Six Flags. And I don't give a whit what people think. When you don't have to be at work until eight in the evening, there's no excuse for oversleeping. But believe me, I still do—most nights of the week, in fact.

Although I hate exercise, I have tried it. (You can stop laughing now. It's true.) I've joined gym after gym and even stayed with it diligently for up to six months at a time. And I never lost a pound. I didn't gain any either, but that's not what I consider progress. After all that blood, sweat, and tears, I didn't look any better and

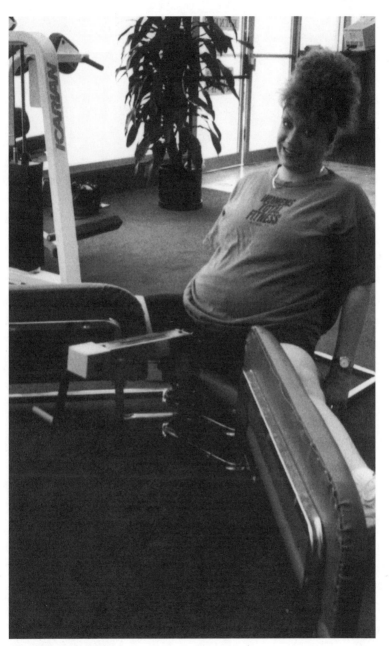

Vaginas of steel.

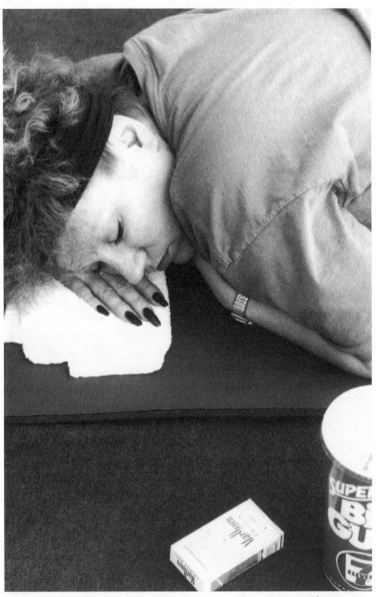

After my workout. (Okay, before—hey, my tacos have to digest! Or I'll get a cramp.)

I sure as hell didn't feel any better either! I was just as hungry and just as ticked off all the time.

The bottom line, however, is that all those things everyone tells you about exercise are <u>not true</u>. People always say, "The hard part is getting to the gym. Once you get there it's easy." What a bunch of crap! Once you get there, it sucks! It is difficult, frustrating, and embarrassing—and that's just talking to the dipsticks that work there. I can't believe the level of morons who work at most of these places. I mean, the towels they carry around are smarter than they are.

Being at the gym was always horrible for me, until the last time I got on the treadmill. Something was different, but we'll talk about that later. As it turned out, Dorothy, you had the power to get home all along, But if I had told you, you never would have found out about it on your own.

Remember, the remote control is God's way of saying, "Relax, let technology do the work for you."

GOING TO THE GYM

Nothing in the world is funnier to me than going to the gym. Mine happens to be an all-women's gym and all the girls there have their makeup done to the nines and their hair done up with BOWS. I've got to say, I don't really get the point of all this, since the gym is ALL

WOMEN. I mean, exactly who are these people getting all prettied up for, anyway?

Fortunately, at my gym (The Women's Total Fitness Center) the "thermometer girls," as I like to call them, are in the minority. That's why I like the place so much to begin with. Most of the women there are overweight and we have a great time. In fact, this is the only gym I have ever been to that I can even tolerate, much less like. And I do like the place, probably because even the women who work there aren't perfect. (To keep the customers from feeling totally sensory-deprived, Jim—the owner—walks around in bicycle shorts, looking like he stuffed a yam down his pants, so at least there's one guy to look at.)

Lisa is my aerobics instructor. I know you all hate the "A" word, and I do too. But let me just say that I am the most uncoordinated person on the planet. I am never in step, I'm always going the opposite direction, and I stop to lie down about every three minutes. And they still don't care!

Most gyms I've been to (in the past) are run by militant psycho women who stare at themselves in the mirror the whole time they're teaching class. What I want to know is, how many hours can you stare at yourself before you pretty much know what you look like? Are they memorizing every single line and wrinkle? Is there going to be a pop quiz later? Will it be multiple choice or essay? Do I need to bring a number-two pencil? I've seen some of these women, and they're positively scary.

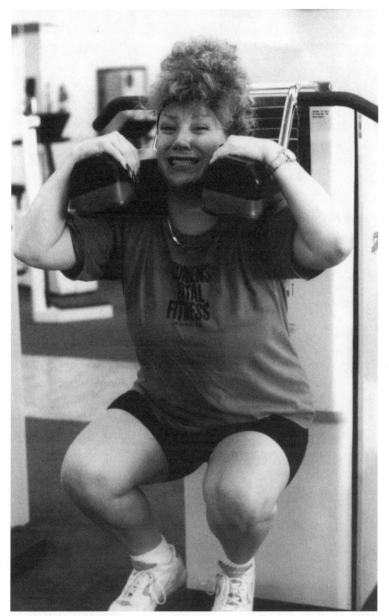

There's one other place I make this face, but only when I skip my Bran-ola!

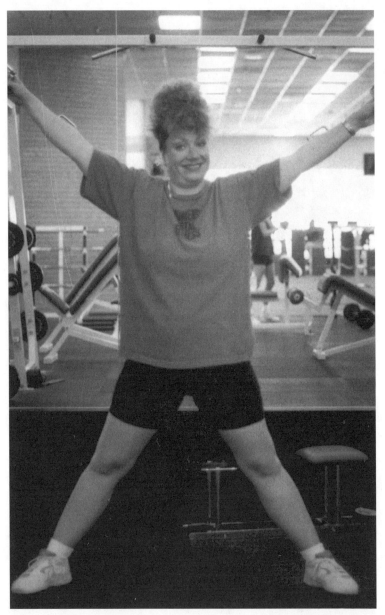

The ONLY way to stand, or lay, without your rolls show-ing—the Starfish position!

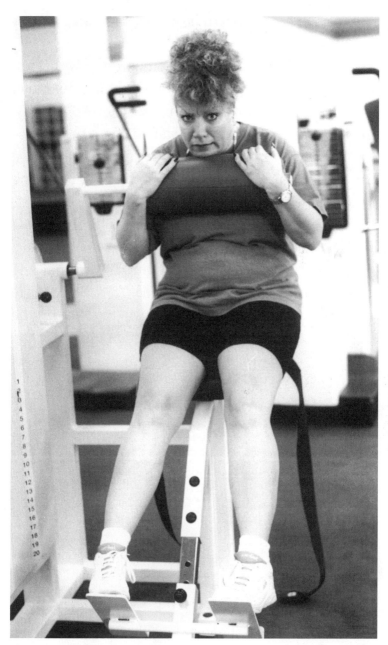

Are you SURE I'm doing it right?

They have these tiny, hard boobs that are going to look like big, floppy clown shoes in about ten years.

But I actually don't mind doing aerobics with Lisa, because she really makes the whole thing bearable. First of all, Lisa isn't your typical instructor—physically, that is. She's actually a little, well, hippy. (There goes that friendship.) But she moves like lightning. I do give Lisa a lot of crap about the things she yells to us during class, but I mean it in a good-natured way.

One of Lisa's meanest tricks is to yell out, "Only eight more! Eight! Seven!" and then she launches into a big, long story that's ten hours long. After that she reads us a couple of chapters of *Moby Dick*. Once that's through, she finishes the countdown, so that by the time we're finished, we've actually done 3,500 of the damn leg kicks instead of just eight. "ARE YOU SWEATING YET?" Lisa also likes to wait until we've been working out for about thirty minutes before she says, "Okay, are you ready to get started?"

But all in all, my gym really does a great job. You may not be so lucky, but my advice to you is to do what I did: Find a place where the instructors aren't fanatics, and where the other members are a little overweight. Going to an all-women's gym takes off a lot of pressure. You can leave the bows at home!

EXERCISE EQUIPMENT

The treadmill is just about the only exercise machine I have been able to cope with. It produces the quickest

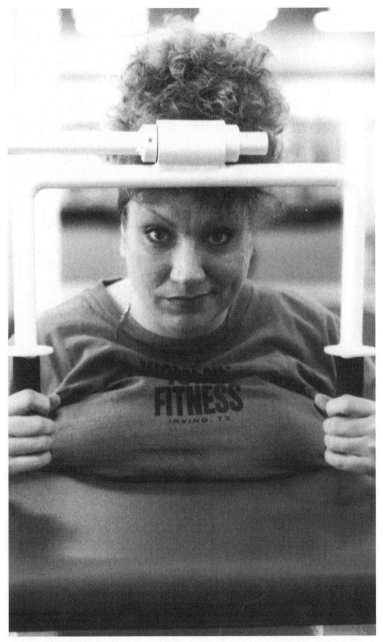

Would you like that chicken with breasts or thighs?

results, but if you're going to maximize your treadmill workout, you have to know the big secret: MUSIC, MUSIC, MUSIC! I can't stay on the treadmill for more than two minutes if I don't have my headphones on. All I do is put on my favorite tape and before I know it, I've been going for thirty minutes. Believe me, I wouldn't lie to you. The time really does go by that fast.

As far as I'm concerned, you can forget the Stairmaster. After about eight seconds on the damn thing, I feel like taking my own life. Plus, there's no ashtray on it, so what's the point?

As for the other exercise machines, I think they're all just ridiculous. I'm sure you agree.

EXERCISE GADGETS

When it comes to exercise gadgets, don't bother, because they don't work. I have two Abdominizers that are still unopened—I got winded trying to open the box—a Thighmaster in the kitchen for opening jars, and a stair-stepper that has three plants on it. (I remember being POSITIVE that I would use the stepper because I could do it in front of the TV, but the couch was always in my peripheral vision, so all I ended up doing was lying down.) I've also bought countless leg and arm weights, but I always lose them when I go swimming.

I also tried one of those new E Z Gliders that you skate back and forth on. Its only problem is that whenever you use it, you can look down and see your reflection. I'd just end up being grossed out.

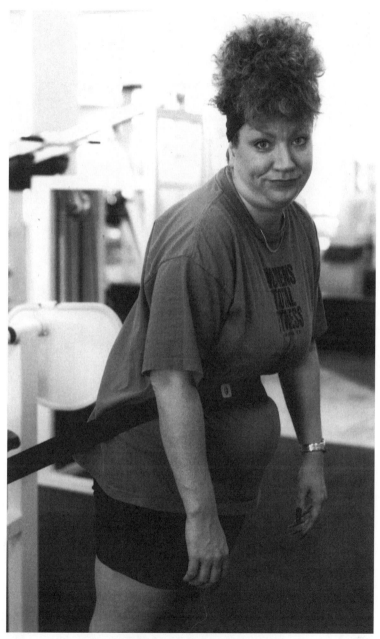

Time for a cold shower, boys!!

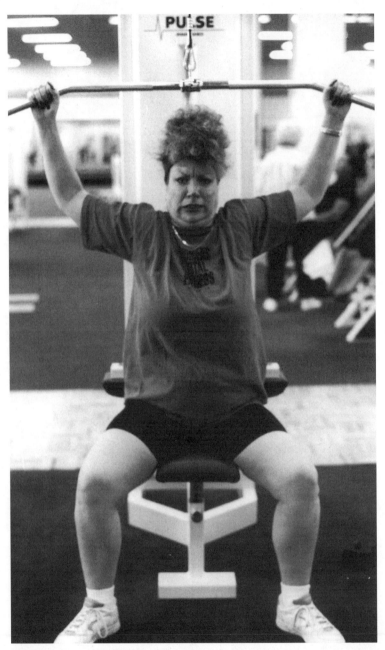

My clothes still fit this hanger.

It was so bad, I had to quit. In the end, I decided it was safer that way. Once I slid so hard I knocked off one of the end blocks and flew through a plate glass window. Plus, the laws of physics tell us that friction can start a fire. With so much weight sliding back and forth, I was going to have to call the fire department each time I used the thing, and I couldn't really afford asbestos socks.

I did try the Thighmaster. Once. But it got stuck. The good news is, I was always ready for a visit to the gynecologist. Unfortunately, it's hard to attract a man when you look like you just got off a horse.

As far as I'm concerned, none of these things are exercise machines, they're toys. Nothing you buy through a television infomercial is going to help you lose weight—except in your wallet.

THE REWARDS OF EXERCISE

The only good thing about going to the gym or partaking in any other form of exercise, is that you feel good afterward . . . sort of. You've given yourself such a good workout and burnt off all those calories—at least three or four—that you feel like you deserve some sort of reward. So that's what I do. As soon as I'm finished at the gym, I think it's only right that I buy myself a little something to make me feel better.

If you've read this far, then I think you'll be able to guess exactly how I reward myself. That's right: FOOD! Since my gym doesn't have one of those chi-chi

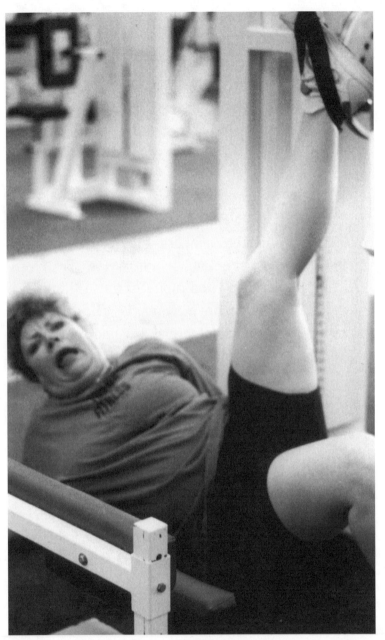

Next stop, Dallas Cowboys Cheerleader tryouts.

snack bars where they charge $15 for a glass of raspberry-beet juice, I usually stop for something to eat on the drive back to my apartment. It's hard to choose between fast food and the supermarket—where I can get something really decadent. But let me tell you, these are the tough decisions you just have to face when you're a grown-up.

I usually opt for the fast food, and not just because I'm lazy. Sure, those drive-through windows are the best invention since the Fry Daddy, but that's beside the point. Actually, I usually choose fast food because it's so much more sinful (which means that right after working out is the best time to eat it. There's less guilt involved then, and that's the whole point of working out, isn't it?)

Living in Texas, you can get so much cheap Mexican fast food down here that you really can't afford not to eat it. So after a good, long workout—in my case, at least seven minutes—I usually stop for a few tacos. I highly recommend it. I will, however, offer you one piece of advice: Try not to eat the tacos while you're driving. It's very difficult and definitely not for amateurs.

OTHER FORMS OF EXERCISE

One of the bigger exercise crazes these days is line dancing. I don't know if you're familiar with it, but it's pretty ridiculous, sort of like redneck aerobics. (If you don't know what line dancing is, count your lucky stars.

It probably means that you're one of the few people who don't have The Nashville Network as part of your basic cable package. If this is the case, you should write your local cable operator and thank him profusely.)

The thing about line dancing is that it just looks absurd. Now, I don't want to make any enemies, but for my money, it's pretty hard to tell the difference between line dancing and activity hour at the state mental hospital. And when I say that, please understand that it's an insult to the mental patients. I know, I've been one.

Not only does it look stupid, but there's absolutely no way that I'm coordinated enough to slap my heel and smile at the same time. Trust me, it's pretty hard to count steps if you can't see your own feet. To make matters worse, it's pretty hard to figure out how much money the guy you're dancing with makes.

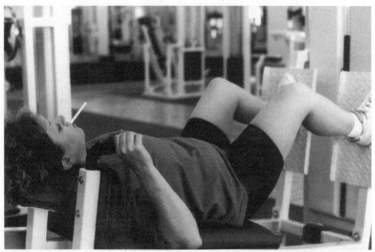

Am I in the wrong office?

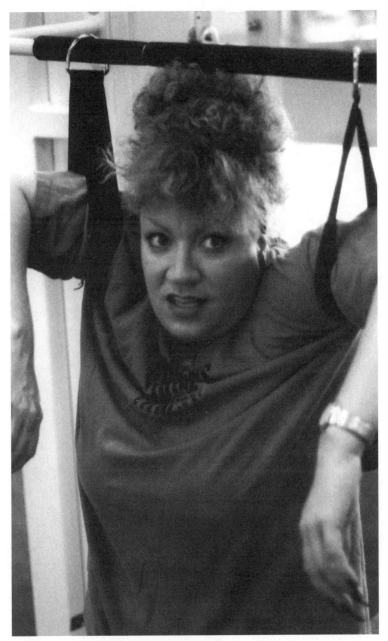

This is the worst ride at Six Flags.

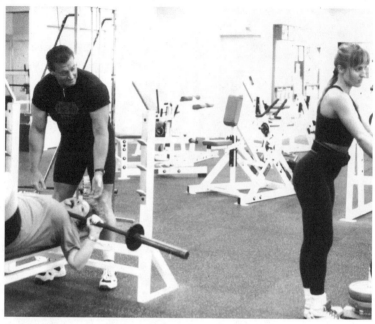

I wanted you to spot <u>me</u>, not her, Conan!

In other words, if I don't know how much money Billy Joe Jim Bob has, I don't know how much breakfast I can order when the club closes. But don't worry, I have the perfect technique to get around this: when you and Billy Joe Jim Bob are dancing, reach over, grab his wallet (hopefully it's not on a chain!), and dump the contents all over the dance floor. If he gets suspicious, just act like you were having a seizure and you couldn't help yourself.

Some people say that to be healthy, all you have to do is eat, breathe, move. That's crap. I say eat, chew, nap.

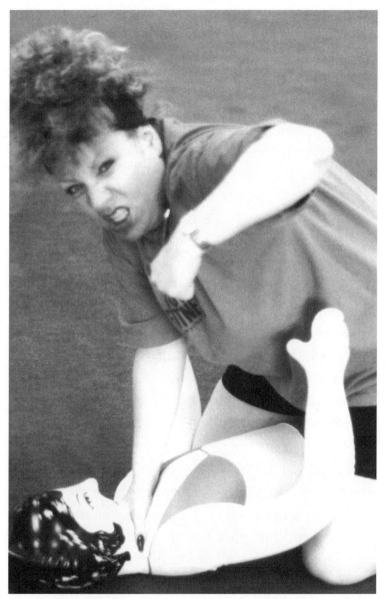

Here's how to "Stop the Insanity!" (For best effect, picture your own doll or dummy with a blonde buzz cut and big mouth!)

Meditation

Of course, exercise and doctors don't work for everyone. (Like me, for example). You and I both know how awful they can be, but there is an alternative. In fact, that's the key to my method: there are always alternatives, so you can always avoid whatever you don't want to do. Some people call this denial. I call it being realistic.

Over the last few years, many people have come to realize that Western medicine and religion don't have all the answers to our problems. That's why so many people have turned to the ancient Eastern religions for alternative ways of coping with the modern world. (Don't worry, I'm not talking about acupuncture here. The only needle I want near my body is the one they use to sew up the turkey on Thanksgiving.)

No, what I'm talking about is meditation, the relaxation technique in which you induce yourself into a trance-like state by clearing your mind of all unnecessary thoughts and focusing your consciousness on nothingness. Meditation was invented by Buddhist monks in Tibet, those guys with shaved heads and long, flowing robes who walk around chanting to themselves. I know this sounds ridiculous to you, but trust me, meditation works. After all, these monks aren't that different from your average fat person, who also wears baggy, loose-fitting clothes and walks around in a trance muttering and trying to find free food.

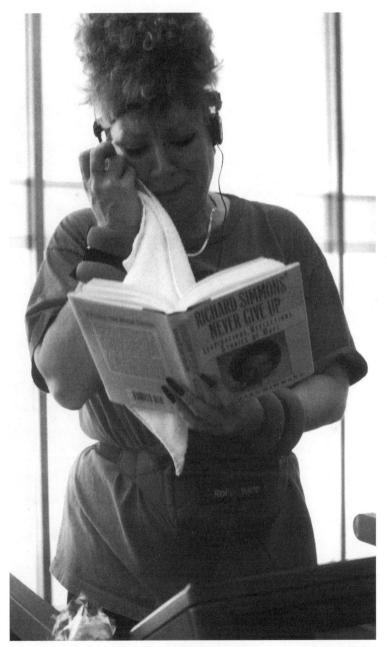

How <u>does</u> he fit into those shorts? (I love you, Richard!)

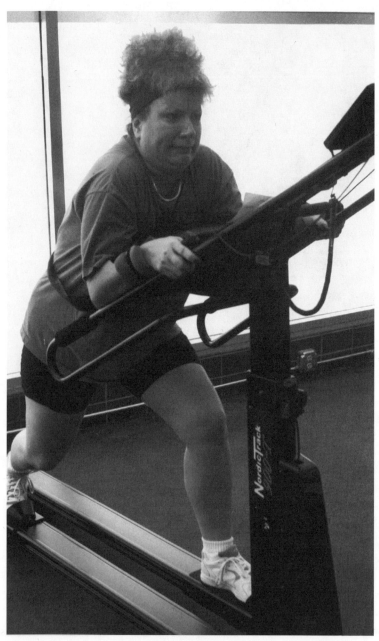

Is this the part where you "really start to feel good"?

The only real difference is that the monks aren't chanting, "Where are the corn dogs? Where are the corn dogs?" but I think you get the picture.

The same way that exercise and dieting are supposed to cure your physical ills (yeah, right!), meditation focuses on soothing your spiritual needs. I know this may sound weird to a lot of you, but trust me, it works. There is no better way to clear your mind of impure thoughts and to put yourself at ease, especially when you're struggling with your weight. (I figure if I tell myself this enough, I'll start to believe it.)

There's an old Buddhist saying that goes, "Free the mind and the body will follow." Of course, my body moves so slowly, it takes about three days for it to catch up, but that's another problem. Basically, you can put a cheeseburger on a stick, and I'll follow you anywhere. The following visualization exercise is an introductory lesson in meditation. Try it. I bet it will work for you if you can stop thinking about food long enough to sit still.

A VISUALIZATION EXERCISE

First, find a comfortable place to sit down on the floor and cross your legs, if you can. I can't, so I usually find some place where I can lie down and relax, like next to the refrigerator.

Now, visualize that first time you saw a fast-food restaurant. Drink in the memories. Picture yourself standing there, staring up at the huge twirling bucket of chicken, knowing your life will never be the same.

As you go further into your relaxed state, reach back into your memory and smell the fried chicken. As the smell curls out of the Colonel's specially designed cooking oven, you know that a single glass door is all that stood between you and your first love, that golden, crispy chicken leg. How could you have known what other treasures awaited—baked beans, cole slaw, and, oh my god, the rolls, the biscuits, the honey, the butter?

Go deeper. Remember the day you turned 16, the happiest day of your life, because you could finally apply there for your first job. Remember how the manager said you would be "sick of chicken within 10 days." You smiled, because you knew in your heart that he could never know the absurdity of that statement. Then you bet him $50 that he was wrong. He still owes you the money.

Go deeper. But at the same time, let go. Remember that after five days you had artfully mastered the skill of slipping your hand between the chicken rack and the tray of "crispies" without getting burned. Think about the secret delight of your first Chicken Deal. Remember meeting the cook after work, outside the back of the restaurant, and exchanging a ten-dollar bill for a shoe box full of crisp, golden chicken. (Do not be ashamed if at this point your meditation becomes a sexual fantasy. Whatever you are feeling is okay. Go with it.)

As you continue on your journey, do not be afraid to recall bad memories as well: the time they told you the bad news, that the skin was the worst part of the chicken and could kill you; the day someone told you the horrible lie that turkey was JUST LIKE CHICKEN, only better for you; and that awful morning when you were fired because they caught you bathing in the baked beans before the store opened. These negative thoughts are an integral part of your spiritual development. You must move beyond them if you are going to make progress.

Now that you are in the deepest part of your unconscious, find your center. Try not to let the gentle humming of the refrigerator motor distract you. Use it to focus your mind. Think about dessert.

Try to maintain this state for 30 to 40 minutes. For beginners, this will be difficult, so don't be afraid to stop at any point in the exercise and have a snack.

This concludes the introductory course in meditation. The advanced course is pretty much the same except you will imagine that you actually marry Colonel Sanders, and you always have to have a supply of Speed Stick "Rotisserie Gold" scent on hand! Actually, with the old Colonel gone, I find myself traveling to Kentucky on the anniversary of his passing, and throwing myself on his grave, sobbing openly. May he rest in peace.

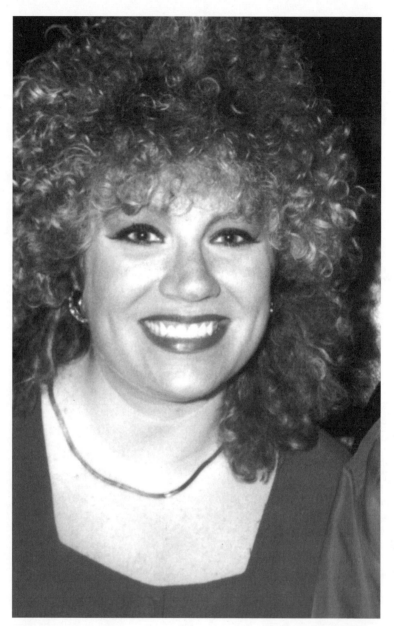

My face has <u>never</u> been fatter... here's your date, The Great Pumpkin!

NINE

There's So Much of Me to Love

They do make lingerie for fat women. In fact, my favorite place to buy it is at a store called, Who Are You Trying to Kid?

ROMANCE

The worst dating tip I ever got was when a friend said to me, "Listen, Beth, there's a club you can join that's full of men who only like fat women." After I finished telling the guy why he was now my ex-friend, I told him why a club full of guys who love fat women just isn't going to solve any of my problems—although just the mention of it did help me remove one annoying person from my life. First of all, I don't want to join a club of chubby chasers to meet Mr. Right. Groucho Marx once said that he wouldn't want to join any club that would have someone like him for a member. That goes double for me when it's a club where the entrance exam involves the scale they use to weigh 18-wheelers and the club crest has a knife and fork on it. Call me old-fashioned, but somehow I just don't think a fat person's club is where it's at.

Second, I know that deep down inside, underneath all these layers, I don't want a man who's attracted to me because I'm fat, mainly because I would have to lose so much weight just to fit into that category. But that's not the only reason I'm against this idea.

If you've read this far, you must think I'm totally obsessed with men and finding one. I've only had two long-term relationships in my life. (Two years is about as long as I can trick a guy into thinking I've got my life together.) But I am 32 years old and my biological clock is ticking. I've hit the snooze bar about as many times as you can, so I'm pretty much ready to have some kids and get the whole thing going. So, yes, I am looking for a husband, but I don't want the kind of man who's going to desire a woman who doesn't think enough to care for her body! In other words, I'm the first to admit that if you're going to attract a guy who isn't just some freak with a fetish for fatsos, you are going to have to do something about your weight.

I guess Groucho Marx was right.

DATING

I remember the first and only time I was rejected by a man because of my weight. It all started when I placed my one and only personal ad in the *Dallas Observer*. I had always sworn I would never do anything so stupid or desperate, so I had to convince myself that I was only doing it to get material for my act. Of course, I secretly hoped and prayed that Dr. Right would answer. At the very least, I hoped one of his assistants would or maybe his missing brother—or someone who hadn't done time. If I was being honest with myself, I would have taken anyone who spoke English.

Here's what the ad looked like:

PERSONAL AD FROM THE *DALLAS OBSERVER*

5'7" SWF seeks SWM. I'm a 31-year-old entertainer (not a "dancer"). You must be emotionally secure because I am in the spotlight a lot. I require a great, dry sense of humor (not "I'm funny at parties"—no lampshades, please). You are 28-38, good shape, mustache O.K., no beards, and not boring.

I think line dancing looks like activity hour at the mental hospital. Your wallet is thick and not on a chain. Professional preferred, but not essential. I'm not a feminist or a man-hater. I have blonde hair, blue eyes, and spectacular fingernails. Big-boned, but not a heifer. I love long walks—IN THE MALL. I hate sports but don't care if you go. Please know how to dress yourself and cut your own food.

I believe you should marry your best friend, not the guy who gives you 50 orgasms. Take me to the state fair! I won't ride the rides, but I love the two-headed goat, and if I don't like you, I'll be dating him next. I only know how to cook three things, but they're great. References available upon request.

NO RUGS, NO DRUGS, NO THUGS

What this means:

I am desperate. I'm a 32-year-old spinster who subjects herself to public humiliation every night in order to meet my bottomless pit of love needs. You must be emotionally secure, because I'm not. You will need enough self-esteem for both of us (I alone count for at least two). You can't be boring because I need you to entertain me 24 hours a day, lest I get bored or have to pursue my own outside interests for a while instead of obsessing about you and our wedding. You are rich and not a redneck. Please have a job.

As for myself, I am a physical monstrosity, but I like to think that great fingernails make up for that. Support me totally, and if you do, you may leave the house on Sunday to go watch a football game with your friends—provided you bring me a present when you come home. Sex will bore me after three months, so you'd better have a good personality. I want to eat out every night. As for the state fair, I really do think it's a nice place for a date: we may not have fun, but there's always the chance that I'll win an agricultural prize.

If you can complete a sentence, I will date you.

I got about 30 letters back. Of course, there really wasn't any material there—they were all really nice letters. I only called one of the guys. Even though he was really sweet, I could tell right away that he wasn't for me—because he was in A BAND. You see, I've been in bands before, so it only took me about 20 seconds to figure out that this guy made about $15.00 a week and lived in his parents' garage. Sorry, but I'm too old to support somebody.

THE BIG NO-NO

If you are fat, single, and lonely, there is one thing that you must NOT do. I don't care if they offer you a free meal at your favorite restaurant and it's going to be served by Kevin Costner in the nude. Under no circumstance should you <u>ever</u> watch *Sleepless in Seattle* alone. A few months ago in Canada, I somehow convinced myself that I could make it through this movie without having a breakdown—I swear it wasn't because the video store was giving out free microwave popcorn with every rental.

So I rented the damn thing and it turned out to be the biggest mistake of my life. I'd been single for about two years, and boy did that movie ever rub it in. After I finished watching it, all I could do was throw myself on the bed and cry my eyes out. Then I burrowed down into the chicken wing bones and started praying. I begged God to send me someone, but He just laughed.

I swear, if the movie studio had any sense of decency, they would put a warning label on the *Sleepless in Seattle* box that says, "Do not watch this movie if you are old, fat, or lonely, or all of the above."

MY BLIND DATE

About a month had passed since I had received the last of my replies. When I got back to Dallas, there was a lone letter in my mailbox from someone who had seen my ad. The letter was from a guy named Craig* (*this name <u>might</u> have been changed to protect the guilty) and it was absolutely hysterical. Craig had also enclosed a picture of himself. He wasn't exactly a dreamboat, but then again, he didn't look like he was storing human heads in the refrigerator either. I thought he was terribly cute.

After the emotional trauma that the damn movie had put me through, I thought, What the hell, and I called him. I could tell he was just my type. For the next two weeks, we talked three and four times a day. Of course, he kept asking me what I looked like, so I told him I was, well, maybe a little overweight. A man would rather hear you'd been in prison than hear this, so then he had to ask exactly how overweight I was.

"Well, can you fit in an airplane seat?" he finally demanded.

"Coach or first class?" was my response.

It got to the point where I had no choice but to send him a photo, so I mailed him my promo picture, which was about 50 pounds old, and told him I was "a little heavier" now. When he asked me how much heavier, I just broke down and lied. I told him I'd been fighting a horrible infection and the doctor put me on steroids for a month. That way, I figured I had a good week to lose 50 pounds before we met for our first date.

The weird thing was, we were having so much fun on the phone that I actually had a flash of self-esteem, a momentary revelation that as of yet has not been equaled again. It only lasted a second, but it was long enough to give me a really stupid idea: THAT IT WOULDN'T MATTER TO HIM WHAT I LOOKED LIKE. By the same token, he was so funny and nice (it's a lot easier on the phone than in person) that by then I didn't care what <u>he</u> looked like. We agreed to meet in Miami, where I was performing, and he had business there. An omen!

Well, the big day came, and I can't ever remember being so nervous. I made my best friend Brian come along and help me pick out an outfit. Then I went and had my hair done. I was supposed to meet Craig in the lobby of the Mayfair Hotel. (I figured that had to be big enough to contain the both of us.) I made Brian come along, too. I figured it was safer, just in case Craig turned out to be the type of serial killer with a great phone personality. But I also wanted Brian there to be a look-out, so he could say THE SECRET PASS-WORD whenever he caught my neck going into double-chin overdrive.

See, I have this borderline double-chin that doesn't show as long as I'm craning my neck (I promise). But whenever I laugh, I turn into Alfred Hitchcock. Since Craig is so funny, I was doomed. Brian and I decided the secret password would be "teacups."

The date went pretty well, even though Brian was yelling "teacups" every five seconds, with Craig asking, "What the hell is teacups?" I thought that everything was kosher. But then again, I also thought I looked pretty good. As you can see from the photograph at the beginning of this chapter, I was stuck inside a very big denial bubble.

At the end of the night, we were saying good-bye, and I was feeling a little tipsy and a lot bold, so I said something brilliant along the lines of, "So, are there sparks for you, too?" He just said, "No." I have never been so stunned in all my life. We'd had so much fun, so of course I wanted to know what had happened. The truth was, he just couldn't get past my weight, literally.

I was devastated. I cried for a week. Couldn't eat—for once! But at least I lost three pounds. All my friends told me Craig was a jerk and a loser. (Maybe not in so many words, but that was the gist of it.) And they all thought I should tell him so. But you know what? I don't agree with them.

The truth, whether you want to hear it or not, is that THERE IS NOTHING WRONG WITH A FIT, HEALTHY MAN WANTING THE SAME IN A MATE. This particular man wanted a woman who took care of herself and it was obvious to him that I didn't. That doesn't make him a jerk. It makes him crazy, but not a jerk.

On the brighter side, at least the story has a happy ending. Craig and I stayed friends, and I've since discovered that he's a complete lunatic, a control freak, and a pervert who no woman on earth would be able to satisfy. He will also make a date with anyone who sounds cute on the phone, so if you're ever on one of those party lines in the Miami area, watch out. But Craig also made me face some facts about myself in his own sick, twisted way and, for that, I'm grateful.

SEX

I think we all know that when it comes to sex, being fat makes the whole thing very, very difficult. Let's face it, if you're a woman over 30, it's hard enough in this country to find a guy who wants to look at you naked. In fact, once I turned 30, every time I went to my doctor's office, he asked me to keep my clothes on. But if you're carrying around extra tonnage, sex is pretty much impossible. I think you all know what I'm talking about: While he's in the bathroom, you're frantically trying to find new and creative ways to lie on the bed so that none (or at least as few as possible) of your fat rolls show.

While there's no easy way to solve this problem, other than losing the 250 extra pounds you're carrying around, I do have one recommendation, a technique that I have developed through rigorous laboratory testing followed up with actual field studies. It's called the "starfish" position; unless you're on your stomach, then I call it "The Little Skydiver." (Little?!)

In the end, we all know that there are only so many ways that you can seductively slide that muumuu down your shoulder.

DISCLAIMER

At this point, I think you know how I feel about exercise (I hate it) and that when it comes to exerting myself physically I'm totally opposed to it unless it's on the jungle gym outside a fast-food place. But just so you don't think I am a total couch potato, I want to leave you with one caveat: You should avoid any and all forms of exercise unless you happen to meet Dr. Right. If you do, FAKE ANY AND ALL PHYSICAL ACTIVITY UNTIL HE MARRIES YOU! Then you can jump back on the couch with the Cheetos and stay there until he divorces you. Once he does, take all his money and go have all your fat sucked out by a plastic surgeon.

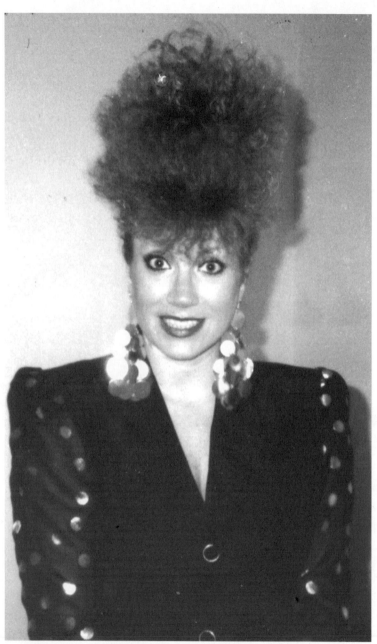

Young Marge Simpson (skinny Beth Donahue).

TEN

Tricks of the Trade

If you're too fat to leave the house, that just means you don't have to take out the trash. Or mow the lawn. Let someone else do it.

First of all, being "fat and jolly" is just a stereotype, and we all know that stereotypes aren't true. (Okay, okay, some of them are, like Japanese tourists carrying cameras, rednecks living in trailers, and clowns crying on the inside.) Sure Willard Scott may seem happy, but that's just because of what they put in his coffee. I don't know that many fat people who are really happy with the way they look, so don't tell me you're "perfectly happy" weighing 300 pounds. You're lying. Maybe you've "accepted" your weight, but don't ask me to buy "happy."

BODY IMAGE

These days, any time you pick up a woman's magazine, all you see are articles about "body image." You can't escape these articles, which is a shame, because the image of my body is the one thing I'm constantly trying to forget. These articles always say that society and the media make women too self-conscious about their looks, because all they do is show pictures of scantily clad supermodels. "Duh!" I always want to say to the editors. "The reason I'm so self-conscious about my body is that you have Cindy Crawford on your cover every month!"

SURVEYS

Some of these women's magazines try, they really do. And just so they can make it seem like they really do care about how we feel about ourselves, they always give us some sort of survey to fill out and send back to the magazine so they'll know what "women like you and me are thinking." Of course, if the magazine editors were really in touch with how American women think and feel, the only survey question they would ask would be exactly how we'd like to see Cindy Crawford killed.

These surveys aren't really scientific or anything, but they do accomplish two things for the magazine. First, they reveal what women just like you and me are thinking—or so the editors would like to believe. Second, they give the editors something to publish instead of another article about how to spice up your relationship or another fun and exciting recipe for Jell-O. For my money, they ought to just combine the two and print an article on how to spice up your relationship by covering yourself with whipped cream and Jell-O.

Sure, women's magazines always tell us that it doesn't really matter how we think and feel about ourselves. But if that's really true, why do they go to such great lengths to figure out how we think and feel about ourselves? In the time it takes the cashier to ring up my food, I usually can read two or three magazines cover to cover, plus a whole *Time-Life* series. Here's a survey I saw recently when I was flipping through a magazine at the supermarket check-out line:

1. "What kind of swimsuit will you wear this year?"
I didn't like any of the choices—string bikini, bikini, French-cut one-piece—so I just wrote in, "the kind with a skirt."

2. "Could you be convinced to wear a bikini in public?"
NO. But then again, I don't think the public could be convinced to look at <u>me</u> if I was wearing a bikini.

3. "What will you do to make yourself look better in your swimsuit this summer?" Please describe your plan in detail.
Call Dr. Kevorkian. No details needed.

4. "What qualities most influenced your decision to buy your last swimsuit?"

Surface area and versatility. If you take it on a camping trip, it will comfortably sleep a family of four.

5. "How do you think you look in your swimsuit?"

Hideous and flabby.

6. "How many swimsuits do you usually try on before you find the perfect suit?"

No human can count that high.

7. "Of which body part are you most self-conscious when you wear your swimsuit: breasts, stomach, hips, butt, thighs?"

All of the above. If you give me a minute I can think of a few more. What about my chin?

8. "Tell us about your most memorable swimsuit experience."

Once, a five-year-old girl surveyed me on a raft and said, "You know, you really look awful in that bathing suit." And I think I heard her mutter the word "Orca" under her breath.

9. "If we need to get in touch with you, where can we reach you?"

Try the nearest Denny's.

Pretty soon, my boobs are going to need their own pair of clogs.

BREASTS

I've always been lucky in that I have really big boobs. In fact, my chest is pretty much the only thing that keeps me from looking like a pear. For some reason, I never lose weight in my breasts, which is both a blessing and a curse. I'm glad I'll never be flat-chested, but I'm beginning to wonder if perhaps things are getting out of control.

If you're reading this and you don't have a chest, DON'T BE JEALOUS. Let me tell you why: I'm 32 years old, and after suffering through years of yo-yo dieting, I now have *National Geographic* boobs. In about a year, I won't need a bra anymore, just pants with really deep pockets. My posture is shot and I walk around looking like I'm searching for a contact lens on the ground.

Flat-chested women always assume that men love big boobs, but I'll tell you a secret: men like to <u>look</u> at big boobs, and they occasionally like to <u>play</u> with big boobs. But <u>MEN MARRY LITTLE BOOBS</u>. Every guy I've ever talked to about this agrees with me, so little-boob girls, you can relax.

If you're fat and have no self-esteem, NEVER go to this restaurant, "Hooters." The last time I was there, I couldn't find the waitress. Finally, I looked behind the napkin holder. "Oh, there you are," I said.

SELF-ESTEEM

My old friend and biggest enemy is Mr. Self-Esteem. He avoids me like the plague. If you're like me, you're sick and tired of hearing about how self-esteem is the key to improving yourself, but at the same time, if you're like me, you'd like to have just a touch of self-esteem for about five minutes so:

1. You'll know what it feels like,

and

2. You'll know what you're shooting for.

I'll tell you right up front, that when it comes to this subject, I haven't a <u>clue</u>. I didn't <u>lose</u> my self-esteem, because I never <u>had</u> it. The psycho nuns beat it out of me with rosary beads in first grade. No lie. That's right, folks, you're on your own with this one. All I can do is tell you that all the self-esteem exercises they try to teach you are nothing but crap. If you don't believe me, look at the following exercise, which I keep taped to my bathroom mirror at home.

<u>**Beth's Positive Affirmations:**</u>

1. Today I will give myself a gift, something no one else would buy me.

That's easy: Pizza!

2. Today, I will pamper myself in some way that I wouldn't normally.

Maybe I'll get out the Garden Weasel and try to shave my legs.

3. Today I will look in the mirror and say, "I am a good, lovable, valuable member of society, and people like to be around me."

First of all, I'm valuable to society because I help keep the food chain going and because I personally keep open eight fast-food franchises that employ a total of 120 people in the Dallas-Fort Worth area. Second, people who weigh 225 pounds like to be around me because I'm five pounds heavier than they are.)

4. Today I will tell myself, "You look pretty" five times.

In other words, today I will get new glasses. In about an hour.

5. Today I will not hurt myself in any way.

Unless I cut myself on the jagged edge around the top of a bucket of chicken.

I think you know the rest of the story. If you've never been taught self-esteem, it's pretty hard to learn when you're 32 years old. You don't believe me? Well, then you are a worthless human being who is doing nothing on this planet but using up everyone else's oxygen! But don't worry, I can relate to that feeling too.

Of course, when I'm thin, my self-esteem isn't so bad. But believe me, I can always find other ways to sabotage it. There is one way I've found that will build self-esteem, but I'll tell you about it later. Well, okay, here it is: Eat nothing but fruits and vegetables!

I know that's not exactly the answer you were looking for.

My best friend Brian and I went to Hawaii. He refused to buy me a muumuu because he was afraid I would grow into it.

FASHION TIPS

Tried and true, here are some of my favorite and best-loved fashion tips. Remember, all of these are doctor-approved, laboratory tested, and guaranteed to make going out in public a little less humiliating:

• Rule Number One—ALWAYS WEAR BLACK. Learn it, follow it, live it: If you're fat, it's the only thing you really need to know about clothes. Always wear black! Always! Your closet should look like a darkroom. I don't know how much simpler I can make it, but you absolutely must remember this rule. There is no other color that can flatter you.

• Broad floral prints are at the top of the no-no list. If you're wearing one, there's a good chance someone will mistake you for a sleeper sofa and sew a doily onto each of your arms.

• Although it's nice to dress like a normal person, I recommend you stay away from jeans as much as possible. The big problem with jeans is that you really can't avoid those creases that form where your thighs connect with your body. Instead of jeans, I recommend palazzo pants. The legs are gigantic and they don't have a waist, which means—you guessed it—no creases!

• If you really want a good scare, take a look at your jeans after you step <u>out</u> of them—if you can, that is. I usually can't, so I have to hook myself up to the garage door opener to pull myself out. When you look down into your empty jeans, you'll probably say to yourself, "There is no way on the face of this earth that my butt can be that big." Believe me, there is. My empty jeans look like the Grand Canyon. In fact, senior citizens book tours to ride through them—with a trail ride to take them down to the bottom. Plus, the county just told me that they're thinking of opening a water park in there.

• If you decide that you absolutely, positively <u>must</u> wear jeans, the first problem you'll be confronted with is how to get into the damn things, (By the way, this is a problem that plagues ALL women, not just us fatties. I don't know why, but even skinny little women insist on buying jeans that are 30 or 40 sizes too tight.)

If you're having trouble getting into your jeans, first of all check the label to make sure they're yours—if the label says "The Delta Burke Collection," you've got the right ones. If, after sucking in your gut and putting on three girdles, you still can't get your jeans on, try lying down on the bed and hooking a coat hanger into your zipper. Pull as hard as you can on the coat hanger. If that doesn't work, get the guys from your office who anchor the tug-of-war team at the company picnic to do it for you.

If that doesn't work, stand your jeans up in the yard and jump off your roof into them.

• When buying shoes, stay away from those six-inch skinny heels. Even if you are one of the lucky three people in the galaxy who can actually balance yourself on these fashionable stilts, every time you take a step in them, you will get stuck in whatever surface you're walking on. (Most places don't appreciate it when you make a golf course out of their floor.)

• When you're looking for a practical shoe, I recommend anything that comes in gold. Gold is practical because it distracts attention away from your body and focuses it on the ground.

• Avoid bright socks at all costs. They draw attention to your tree trunk ankles.

• When you're looking for pantyhose, there's one thing you need to remember: QUEEN-SIZED IS NOT FOR QUEEN SIZES; it's for women who are coming off anorexia. Ladies, the back of the package IS LYING TO YOU. If you are more than four feet tall and weigh more than 68 pounds, move on to fat-lady hose. Nothing in an egg is going to fit you (unless it's an ostrich egg).

For my money, the best fat-lady hose are called "Just My Size." The sizes are reasonably accurate and they're really durable. (They have to be when your thighs rub together as much as mine do.) They're so durable, that if you're having a dinner party, you can use the panty-hose to strain your pasta and then wear them the same night. How's that for fashion with practicality? The greatest thing about "Just My Size" hose is that if you ever do lose weight, you can use them as a hammock in your backyard.

• MAKE YOUR HAIR AS BIG AS HUMANLY POSSI-BLE. If you can get it wider than your hips, that's a good start. The bigger your hair, the better the chance that you can get that "V"-shaped look going, and this will create the illusion of thinness. (It will still be only an illusion, but it's better than nothing.) Some say big hair is "out" but I don't care. Defy fashion! Make your hair wider than a Winnebago. Tease it. Mousse it. Gel it. Use a pitchfork if you have to. Just get it out there. Curls are a good idea, because they will give your hair volume. Your goal should be to look like an airplane coming in for a landing.

• Never, ever wear your hair in a bun on top of your head. You'll end up looking like one of those Buddha statues, except unlike the Buddha, you won't be at one with the universe. And you definitely won't be smiling. The other big no-no is a short haircut. I know it's hot when you're carrying around more extra baggage than a sky cap, and I know the easiest way to cool off is to get all that hair off your head. But the truth is, if you're fat and you have really short hair, you'll end up looking like a tick.

• Long fingernails and big earrings are good disguis-es. They lend you that spark of femininity you desper-ately need when you weigh more than most other women—and for that matter, most other families. Best

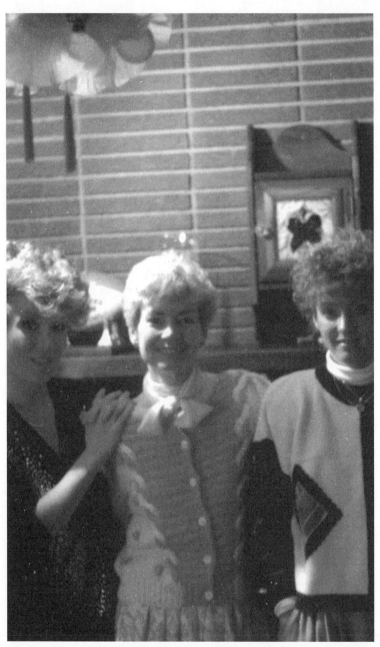

The Donahue Girls (from <u>right</u>) Skinny, Skinnier, and Me!

of all, nice fingernails and earrings make it look like you actually care about the way you look.

For a more complete guide to buying clothes, read on.

BATHING SUITS

Spring is the time when nature blooms again, love is in the air, and every fat person in America starts to miss those lovely winter layers that hide the way you look so nicely. In this season of renewal, nothing renews the knowledge that I'm really, really fat quite like spring and summer fashions.

You and I both know that the worst, the absolute most humiliating and depressing part about being overweight is that first trip to the department store to look at the season's hottest new beach fashions. Of course, the key word there is look, since all those hot new fashions for fun in the sun are designed for stick-figure supermodels and women whose idea of a balanced breakfast is a bowl of Corn Flakes. (Two flakes, that is.) After I finish "looking" at all those string bikinis, strapless tops, and thongs that aren't big enough to be my shoelaces, I send my ego over to the shoe department while I grab a few suits from the new "Barbara Bush Collection" and slink off to a dressing room to face the truth.

The most important rule for bathing suit shopping is the following: If you're really huge, you want a bathing suit that has a skirt. You'll want one from the *Gone With the Wind* collection, complete with hoops. But remember, it must be kept away from children at all times. I still remember being a kid and reaching into the beach bag for candy money and accidentally touching my mom's bathing suit. It was the kind with the fake boob cups and it scared the living daylights out of me.

Just the other day, I was flipping through a magazine and came across an ad for a particular mail order catalog's bathing suits. (I won't tell you which catalog it is, but I'll give you a hint: it's one of those really preppy ones where the models look almost as life-like as mannequins.) Anyway, the ad promised me that I wouldn't "Ever Have to Feel Self-Conscious at the Beach Again." Since that sounded too good to be true, I thought I better take a closer look. Here's what I found:

1. Their suits come in "three different torsos, because a tall woman may have a short torso, a short woman may have a long torso."

That's great, but what if you're Jeffrey Dahmer, and you have them all?

2. Since some women are very well-endowed, their fat-lady bathing suits come with "shelf bras."

What they don't tell you is that some assembly is required and you're probably going to need a hammer, a socket wrench, and—most likely—a subcontractor. But don't worry, it's worth the effort. And you can put your whole *Nancy Drew* collection between your boobs on your new shelf.

3. Their bathing suits are available with special "slimming fabrics."

Guess what, ladies? It's RUBBER! And if you order your suit three sizes smaller than you usually wear, you'll really get a slimming effect, because you won't be able to breathe…YOU'RE DECOMPOSING!

4. Their suits are made of "really durable fabrics."

This means that they hold up well in chlorinated pools, swamps, toxic chemical spills, and, if you're looking for the ultimate workout, quicksand!

5. "The beauty of ordering a bathing suit from a catalog is that you can try it on in the privacy of your own home!"

Now I know you're usually tempted to try the bathing suit on at the flea market or at a major sporting event, but this method is much more convenient. You can be alone—just you, the bathing suit, your mirror, and a chainsaw.

Of course, the ad also promises that once you try on the suit, if you see something you don't like, you'll be able to return it. Does that include my reflection?

One size fits all? All what? Praying mantises? To the best of my knowledge, "One size fits all" is about size 10.

SHOPPING

One of my all-time least favorite things to do when I'm fat is buy clothes. (I mean it! Read my letter at the end of this chapter if you don't believe me.) To begin with, the selection is horrendous: you can always find plenty of styles that look good at home, the office, and the tractor pull. At department stores, it drives me crazy that the fat lady clothes are always downstairs in the basement. They must put us down there, out of view and away from the commotion upstairs, so the brainless sales robots at the makeup counters can concentrate. I guess it must be very difficult to prescribe a pore cleanser when you have a fat person in your line of vision. What are they going to do, slip and recommend Log Cabin syrup?

The only thing worse than being stuck in the basement is when the store puts the "Woman's World" section right next to the "Petites." And they always do. It's bad enough that they won't let you shop upstairs with the normal people, but do they have to put you beside the beanpoles? To their credit, at least this layout makes it easy to tell where your section ends and theirs begins. I admit, however, that I do have trouble sometimes: I once tried to buy a petite knit miniskirt—I thought it was one of those elastic bands that holds up a ponytail.

By the time I hit 235 pounds, I was pretty much locked out of the regular-sized stores. (You know you're fat when you walk into a normal department store and the security guard starts laughing.) At the human-sized stores, the clothes start at size 1-2 and go up to 13-14. The only problem is, the decent clothes start to drop off at about size 9-10. There's about 70 million 3-4s, 5 billion

5-6s, and lots of 7-8s and 9-10s (these figures are approximate, kind of like my figure). Once you get up to the 13-14s, all that's left is one pair of lime green bellbottoms with the zipper ripped out. It's always right next to the shirt with three sleeves. Normally I wouldn't buy something as hideous as lime green bellbottoms, but since they're marked down to $5.00, I'll take 'em! (The three-sleever, by the way, makes a great Christmas present—long johns for your well-endowed boyfriend.)

The bad news is that I'm long past size 13-14. The good news is that since I'm only a size 18-20, when I go to the fat-lady store I'm usually the skinniest chick in the joint! How's that for rationalization? All the other women spend the afternoon there jealously eyeing my one chin and my one fat roll—even if it is ON MY BACK!

What I love about the fat-lady stores is that the names are so discreet. They're always called something like "Queen Mary," "The Forgotten Woman," or "The Missing Link." My personal favorite is, "Lay Off the Butter, Fatty." But like the rest of you, I do most of my shopping at Lane Giant. I do have to give them some credit, because the clothes there are getting a little better—apparently someone just told the company about cotton.

There are two things I like about Lane Giant. First, even though it's not exactly high fashion, at least they have a great selection. There's always plenty to choose from, even if you're a size 88. The other thing I like about the store is that they display their clothes on those giant round silver racks, and on top of each one is a Lazy Susan with chips, dip, party mix, and M&Ms. These people are not stupid—they don't want you to get any thinner!

But what I don't understand about Lane Giant is why they use ISABELLA ROSSELLINI as the model in all of their photographs! I'm not lying—go look! Do they take a photo of her and then use the old "Silly Putty and the comics" trick to stretch the picture out so she looks like you and me? How stupid do they think we are? Just because we let ourselves get this big, it doesn't mean we've lost all our critical faculties. I know the only foreign model car their cover-sized bra is going to make me look like is the Mercedes-Benz station wagon.

I still remember the time I went to Lane Giant with my ex. (Ladies, if you want to lose a man, this is probably the quickest way to do it—other than letting him see you naked.) He was trying to be helpful, so he grabbed something he liked and rushed over to me and said, "How about these, honey? They'd look great on you." "Those are the curtains to the dressing room," I said. "Put them back. Now!" The woman who was changing in there at the time was not amused.

One good thing about the fat-lady stores is the size of the dressing rooms. They are huge—I guess because they have to be. They're big enough that you could play racquetball in there (hey, not that *I* would, but you could.) And they're not just big in Texas, they're big everywhere. One time I was in a fat-lady store in Orlando, Florida, and I got some clothes together, and I went up to the salesperson to ask if I could try them on. She said, "Yes, but don't go in dressing room four. Disney on Ice is rehearsing!"

Recently, after getting a little tired of the clothes at Lane Giant, I thought that maybe I'd try shopping at a department store for a change. So I trucked on over to Macy's, thinking their selection might be a little better. Wrong! What is wrong with designers these days? Most women are at least a little overweight, and just in case no one has noticed, there are millions of fat women in this country. Don't designers realize that they could make millions if they would just make us some decent clothes? Apparently not.

Designers everywhere, please listen to someone who knows: Just make us the same styles you make for skinny people. The same pattern and everything, but in a larger size! If they look terrible on us, then that's our fault for buying them, but at least give us a chance! I swear, if I see one more giant peach tunic with fake appliqués on it, I am going to puke. Quit insulting us. Fat doesn't mean "stupid," it means "hungry"!

The last time I went shopping, I tried about 600 different department stores and did not find a single thing that was the least bit hip or fashionable. Not a single dress had a waist on it. Every one was a giant tent, a big, shapeless monstrosity and SLEEVELESS!

That <u>really</u> pisses me off. Have you ever seen a fat person with skinny arms? Of course not! We all have big, floppy, lunch-lady arms. I haven't worn a sleeveless gown since I was baptized, and if you saw me in one right now, you'd probably want to dunk me in a pool of water, too. So, fashion designers of the world, the conclusion should be obvious: STOP MAKING SLEEVELESS DRESSES FOR FAT WOMEN! We don't wear them, we won't wear them, and we shouldn't wear them. I have never seen a fat woman in a sleeveless dress, but I have seen thousands of dresses that I would buy in a second if they had sleeves. Can you hear me, Calvin Klein?

FASHION FOR MEN

Since I'm not a guy, there's not that much advice I can offer you, except that for you portly fellows out there, form-fitting clothes are a mistake. As far as we ladies are concerned, looser is better. Nothing is more horrifying—except maybe my upper arms—than seeing a really fat guy wearing really tight pants that accentuate the Loch Ness monster-sized bulge around his waist that all fat guys seem to get. I don't know if you need a larger size, pleats, or just a circus tent, but please, gentlemen, please: do not wear pants that show off your Continental Shelf.

Here is a minimally revised version of an actual letter summarizing an actual incident I sent to a Dallas newspaper while I was writing this book. Although the letter didn't get published, it accurately reflects what chubbies like me have to live through:

Never in my life have I been so blatantly discriminated against for being fat than I was last weekend. There is a real fancy-schmancy dress shop here in Dallas I'll call "Witchamacallit." They advertise "Cocktail dresses, stage clothing, beaded tops, pageant gowns, and the best selection for all occasions that always get a second look." I'd seen billboards for this store all over town for years, and after seeing an ad in the paper for an 80-percent-off sale, I decided to make the drive. I had a television appearance coming up and I wanted something sparkly and fun, so I set off. As you know, I didn't really expect it to be a fat-lady store, but these places usually have The Cow Rack shoved over in the corner, offering up a few nightmares to choose from.

On the way to this store, I stopped at a mall, where I combed the BASEMENTS (of course...keep the heifers downstairs, for God's sake!) to check for that once-in-a-lifetime freak of nature dress that occasionally slips through the cracks. No such luck. Same old shapeless tents. They were having a sale: "Get your Dowry from the old folks home for 20 percent off today only!" All right! I trudged up to Old Faithful, Lane Giant (stopping to browse at the Food Court, of course...now THERE'S a selection!), where I bought a couple of things out of sheer desperation, and then I headed on over to "Witchamacallit."

When I walked into the store, I thought I had died and gone to heaven. There must have been—no lie—at LEAST five thousand dresses in this sequin warehouse—shoes, earrings, hats, everything. And for ONCE I had some money to play with. I should have packed a lunch (or two) this place was so big. I was carrying a "CBS Television" tote bag with me, figuring this would improve my chances of getting waited on. (Works every time!)

Sure enough, in three seconds, this twitchy, little anorexic is on me. "Oh my God! Do you work for CBS?" she squeals. I said "Yes" (lie) and kept on walking. I LOATHE to be followed around when I am shopping, and since I knew I was going to be there for hours, I figured I'd better set the rules with her. "That has ALWAYS been my dream!" she said. Really. Well, MY dream is to look around this store without getting impaled by your Mail-bangs every time I turn around. Of course I didn't say that. I told her I was JUST LOOKING and told her

I would come and find her the minute I needed any help... Every time I turned around, there she was, two inches from my face. I finally gave in.

"Okay, where is the fat-lady section?" I asked. Well, you'd have thought I'd just told her that The Gap had just burned down. The look of fear, horror, and revulsion on her face was hysterical. Then she looked around to make sure no one was around and says—and this is a direct quote—"We don't have any. Our owner has very specific feelings about none of the clothes in the store being over size 12."

What!????! Are you KIDDING me?! She went on to say that he just wants to cater to the thin. Now mind you, this girl was not being mean. In fact, to her credit, she looked pretty embarrassed. But she couldn't have been more than 17 years old and just didn't have enough brains to know that there are about 289 different ways to say what she said without saying it that way. It was obvious that she was just repeating what she was told.

I said, "You're kidding me, right? In this WARE-HOUSE you don't have ANY large sizes?" Chewing furiously on her fingernail, she looked alarmingly like Dustin Hoffman in Marathon Man, and conspiratorially drags me over to the Mother-of-the-Bride rack, which looked like the Golden Girls garage sale, and STILL there was only one size 14. YES! A lavender chiffon tunic! Start a LIST of the places I can wear this! I turned to her and said, "You know, maybe if you had some normal sizes in this joint, you wouldn't need to have an 80-percent-off sale!" Blank stare. I then BEGGED her to leave me alone so I could at least look at earrings and shoes. (They didn't even carry my shoe size!!—9 1/2)

She said, "I can't. My manager will yell at me." I looked around and noticed that no one else had a guard dog, and that's when it dawned on me: She was trying to drive me out of the store! I was absolutely STUNNED. As I turned to leave, I got a look at the "owner": He was 400 pounds if he was an ounce!

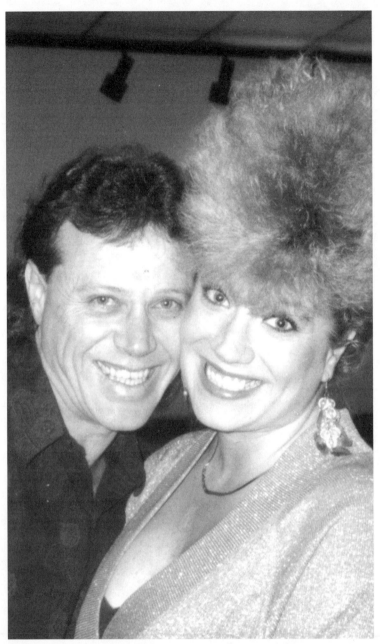

If you use <u>lots</u> of hairspray, he can't get away!!

ELEVEN

Climbing the Mountain — Yourself

I want to move to Los Angeles to get discovered. The only problem is, there's a weight limit on Melrose Avenue.

THE POINT OF IT ALL

By now you're probably saying, "Alright, Beth, enough of the fat jokes. I know I'm fat—I can see that by looking in the mirror. But where's the big message that you've promised us all along?"

Well, kids, here it is.

You've stuck with me this far, so now you get to hear it. But don't worry, I know you're as skeptical about this as I was before it happened to me. Trust me, I've read all the same inspirational crap you have, and I don't buy a word of it. No one else can tell you how to fix your own problems—you basically have to sit down and decide that you're going to take care of them yourself.

It's a protracted, painful process called "bottoming out," and it's usually a very long free-fall that gets you there. Some people never hit bottom, but most of us eventually do. I sure did, and as painful as it was, I'm so glad it happened.

Sometime in early 1994, I was having dinner with a comedy club owner that I hadn't seen in a couple of years. This is when I looked and felt my worst. My weight sure reflected it. I was a mess, and the sad thing was, it had been so long since I'd cared about myself, I didn't even realize how bad I had gotten. The guy I was eating with is one of my staunchest supporters, but once we sat down at the table, he just laid into me. He told me that every guy in the comedy business used to have the hots for me and wanted to know why I had let myself completely fall apart.

Then he really let me have it. He said to me, "Do you really want to be on TV looking like this?" The truth was, I didn't. I had turned down two television appearances because I was so embarrassed about my weight. My friend's diatribe continued, and he was really being mean. But the thing was, we both knew what he was trying to do: He was giving me the slap in the face that no one else had the nerve to give me.

I don't know why the message clicked that time, but it sure did. (Actually, I do know one of the reasons the message clicked: I hadn't had a date in about two years. I mean, no one was looking at me anymore, not even the loser guys that are still at the bar when they turn

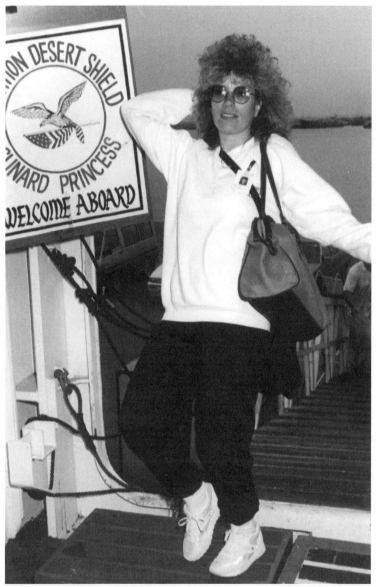

Arriving in Saudi Arabia for the war... 20,000 soldiers and for once I was dating someone. The <u>second</u> I got off the plane back in Texas, I got dumped!

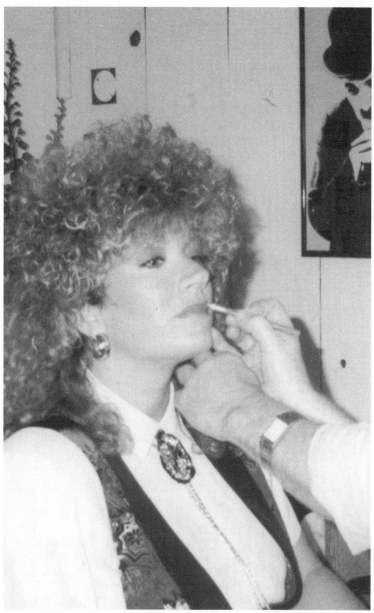

Minutes before my first "VH-1 Stand-up Spotlight"... This is the life.

the lights on at last call.) I had known for a long time that I was getting out of control, but it's amazing how you can still rationalize everything, isn't it? I remember after I got to 175 pounds, I swore that I would never get to 200, and then there I was at 230 saying that I'd never get to 250.

This time, something snapped, and I just knew that I had two choices: keep getting fatter and fatter, until I developed my own atmosphere, which means that I would get even lonelier and more depressed; or do something about it. So I did something about it.

Since I had no intention of giving up my favorite foods—and never will—I knew my only hope was to start exercising. I've already told you how I feel about exercise, so I think you know how hard it was for me to come to that conclusion. It wasn't easy, but I knew I didn't have another choice, so I just decided to take it one day at a time.

In the beginning, my only goal was to not hate it, because if you hate something, you give it too much power. I also knew that I was never going to like it, so I figured I'd just start out taking baby steps. At night I would ask God to please help me get to the gym for an hour. That's all I would do—just ask Him to help get me there. And He did.

Now, I don't know who your god is, but it really doesn't matter. I don't care if it's Jesus, Yahweh, Buddha, Robert Tilton, Richard Simmons, or if you're really desperate, Fabio, but the point is, it's nice to have a little help to get you over that first hump. Alcoholics Anonymous tells you that at some point, if you want to get better you just have to turn yourself over to a higher power. And you know what, they're right. Whether you are a spiritual person or not, you're going to need some help along the way. You just can't do it all alone. And a screaming, bald lady isn't going to work.

I went to the gym every day for three months, and I never lost a pound. I was really frustrated, but everyone I knew said that I <u>had</u> to keep going, that one day the weight would start to come off. Eventually it did. And then the most amazing thing started to happen, something people had always told me about, but I had never believed them: I started not to hate myself. For me, that's the miracle. I'm not going to tell you that I love myself, and I'm certainly not going to tell my priest, but I'm getting there. But then again, for me, just not wanting to throw up when I look in the mirror is a really big step.

The funny thing is, it's not just about the weight anymore. I just know somewhere inside that I'm doing something good for myself that doesn't involve the mall. I know this sounds really trite, and I know that you've heard it all before, but I don't walk the treadmill for 45 minutes every day because I'm losing weight. I do it because each time I do that little workout, it gives me another grain of self-confidence that I haven't gotten in almost 25 years of therapy, pills, doctors, and rehab centers. I don't pretend to know why it works, but then again, I don't care, just as long as it keeps working.

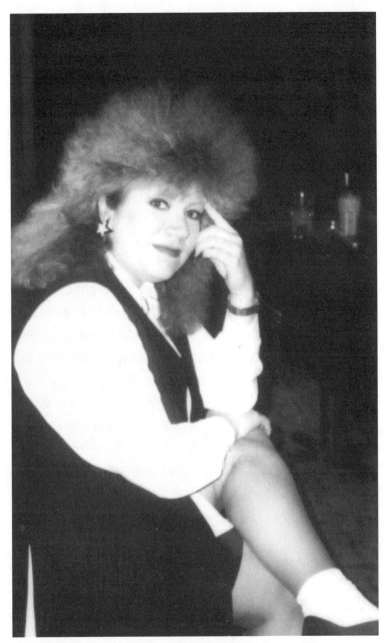

New Year's Eve, 1993-94; Sister Mary Angus Young.

I think the bottom line is that it's all about doing something hard that goes against everything you believe in and everything you ever thought you could do. You don't have to change your whole life, just start with this one thing. I know that everyone reading this book would rather have a little self-esteem than lose weight, but the miracle is that you can have both if you just get your ass on that treadmill (with the headphones, or else it won't work) for 30 minutes just a few times a week. Before you know it, a change that you never thought would happen for you will happen. So get on that treadmill. Or take a walk around the block. Or swim a few laps every day (you can leave out the headphones here—you don't want to electrocute yourself).

And one other thing: Don't try and change your eating habits right away. You'll just feel deprived and resentful, and resentment kills everything.

As for me, well, I'm still pretty huge. I just got under 200 pounds after six months, but I've tasted self-esteem, and I want more. I'm 32 years old, and it's time to quit playing games. I'm an adult, and this fat is not going to come off by itself. And the choice is mine.

It's yours, too. Just try not to hate it.

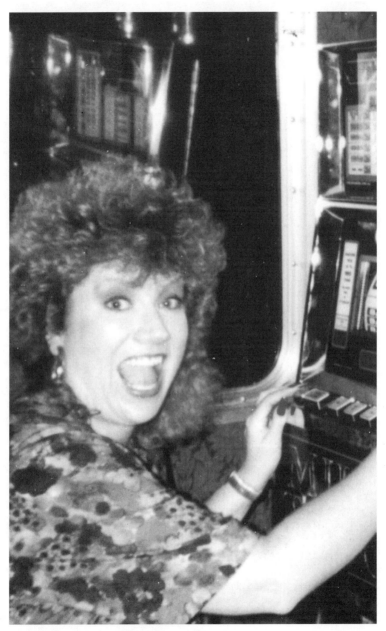

Hey, I just won a cheeseburger!

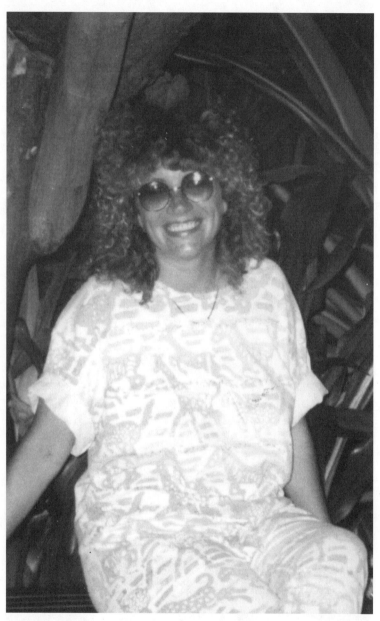

My plunge into Hugeness starts in Hawaii... WHERE'S THE GIFT SHOP?!

TWELVE

Questions and Answers

When people heard I was writing this book, they assumed for some reason that I was some kind of expert on being fat. Couldn't they tell that just by looking at me? It's funny, though, how once people think you're an expert, they'll come up to you at the strangest times and ask for advice. I guess doctors get this all the time at cocktail parties. As soon as someone hears they're an M.D., they immediately say something like, "Oh, really? Could you tell me why I get this sharp pain in my foot every time I get out of bed in the morning?" The answer's usually, "Because your husband spreads broken glass and rusty nails at the foot of your bed."

As a comedian, I'm used to people coming up to me and saying, "Hey, if you're so funny, say something that'll make me laugh." That's when I tell them, "First give me $25, I'm off the clock." (It gets a laugh every time.) But being an expert on weight loss is something entirely different. It's still kind of new to me. So is losing weight, but I think I'm getting the hang of it. I'm also getting used to the kind of questions people ask me. They usually fall into one of three categories: stupid, really stupid, and what time are you due back at the institution?

So, to save you the time of writing me a letter or coming up to me when you see me in the Frequent Customer line at Jack in the Box—and to save me the aggravation of having to deal with people when I'm trying to decide how many cheeseburgers to order—I've decided to print the questions that people ask me most frequently. I'm sure this chapter won't answer all your questions, but hopefully they'll go a long way toward getting me a little more free time when I'm trying to buy food.

Believe me, it's not easy being a guru, but somebody's got to do it.

Q. How often should I exercise?

Exercise whenever you have a date (start three weeks before), when you're having your picture taken for any reason (your driver's license photo would be an exception), or when you're dating a guy who exercises (but only until he marries you—for more information on this rule, see the chapter on exercise).

Q. How many calories should I eat every day?

Never let your caloric intake exceed your white blood cell count.

Q. How much should I weigh?

It varies from person to person, depending on height. According to my weight, for example, I should be 9 feet, 11 inches tall.

Q. Can you ever be too rich or too thin?

You can never be too rich, but you can be too thin. If you are pregnant, and you don't need a sonogram to see your baby, then you're too thin.

Q. What's your favorite kind of food?

My favorite food is anything deep fried. I really took it personally when Kentucky Fried Chicken sold out and changed their name to KFC, as if we're not going to think it's fried just because they changed the name. There is nothing anywhere on this planet more wonderful than fried chicken.

Q. What's your favorite fast-food restaurant?

See above.

Q. How come some fat people have really skinny legs?

Because the food never makes it to their legs. Most people don't know this, but the stomach can act like a Venus Fly Trap, snatching the food before it has a chance to trickle down into the leg area. The overflow usually only makes it to the butt and the upper thighs.

Q. Is Susan Powter nuts?

'Fraid so. She says in her book that she's not in it for the media attention, yet she's on "Circus of the Stars" every three weeks. (And she scares the tigers!) I'm certainly not opposed to making money, but at least be honest about it. You've got to be gentle with people, you can't scream at them. I guess it is possible to shave your head and scare people into eating right, but I question how successful this will be in the long run.

Q. What's the deal with Richard Simmons?

To be honest, he's someone I used to laugh at—until I got fat. My gut feeling (some pun intended) is that he really does care. I wrote him a letter once and got a personal reply within two weeks. I usually have to wait longer to hear back from my own agent, to say nothing of family members. You'd have a hard time convincing me that he's in it for the money. He was huge, he's been there, he knows. I adore him.

Q. How long should I spend at the gym every day?

Add fifteen minutes to the time it takes you to get there and get back home.

Q. Should people be allowed to wear thongs?

Only if you can actually see them.

Q. What's the most important meal of the day?

They say it's breakfast. I hate breakfast. But when it was explained to me in terms that I could understand, I finally saw the light. Sort of. The truth is that your body doesn't work unless you get some fuel in the morning, so now I gag down a small bowl of 10-grain Colon Buster cereal with little or no problem. Of course, I do sprinkle on some Coco-Puffs for added flavor. The best part is, I've finally come to enjoy the pleasure of regular bowel movements without blood-curdling screams coming from the bathroom every eight days.

Q. Do you know a good appetizer that can be prepared in a hurry?

I always recommend chocolate chip cookie dough on a Ritz cracker.

Q. How do you feel about cosmetic surgery?

Once I get the cash, I'm on the table that day. I've got a Sara Lee cheesecake in my right butt-cheek that I need

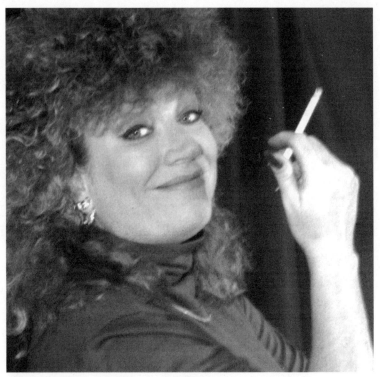

My favorite snack!

to get sucked out because it just won't budge. While he's got me under, I would also appreciate it if the doctor would drain the Alfred Hitchcock chin, lift the boobs, and shrink each nostril circumference by about three inches.

Q. How many calories will I burn off during sex?

Awake or asleep?

Q. What's your favorite diet?

The embalming diet. When you're dead, it doesn't matter anymore.

Q. Are there any diets that do work?

No.

Q. Why does diet food taste like cardboard?

Because they've taken out anything that might be remotely pleasurable to the taste buds so that <u>you won't be able to eat it</u>! Therefore, they're able to proclaim that their diet works!

Q. How long should I wait between meals?

Just long enough for that my-stomach-is-going-to-explode feeling to pass. Once you sense there is one tiny cranny of space in your gut, proceed at your own risk.

Q. What about diet drinks?

They're not bad—as long as you put ice cream in them. As far as diet soft drinks go, I recommend Diet Dr Pepper, and that's it. It's the only drink that doesn't taste like it's diet.

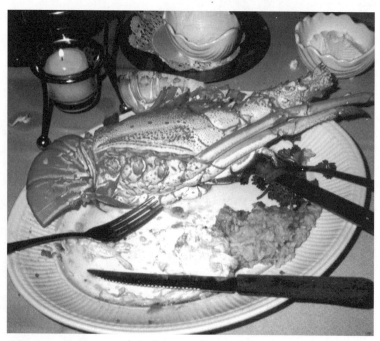

"And we have turned the past into the greatest lobster-fest of them all!"

Q. How do you get a Big Mac stain out of an evening gown?

Don't worry about it. Just tell everybody that your dress was designed by Ronald McDonald. Then point to your French fry earrings as proof.

Q. How much water should I drink?

This is a toughie. My best advice is to stick your head under the sink with your mouth open. Stop right before you pass out or wet your pants, whichever comes second.

Q. What should I use to count calories?

Price Waterhouse.

Q. Do I have to exercise?

Basically, you have two choices. You can eat celery for the rest of your life, or you can drag your butt onto the treadmill three times a week. Sorry, but that's the truth.

Q. What is cellulite and how do I get rid of it?

Cellulite is simply all of the stored popcorn, peanuts, and other food products that make you look like you got shot in the butt with a round of BBs. It doesn't go away—ever—and I will personally choke the life out of anyone who buys that cellulite creme crap. Use spackle.

Q. Do I need to see a doctor before I start exercising?

No. Give me the $45, and I'll tell you the same thing he will. "Go slow. Next!" If you're really, really fat, don't see a doctor, see a priest and have an exorcism.

Q. When it comes to exercise, is it all right if I skip a day?

Honey, you can skip a week for all I care. But it does help if you're Catholic, because then you have enough guilt stored up to get you back in there the next day.

Q. How can I calculate the fat content of my food?

Take your birth date, multiply it by six, divide by the smallest number of pepperoni slices you'll settle for on a pizza. Add to that the number of orgasms you've faked in the last year. This is the fat content of your food.

Q. What do you think of vegetarians?

Anyone who tells you that fish and chicken aren't meat is lying. But if you think it's weird that some people will only eat things that come out of the ground, I have a Jewish friend who won't eat anything that rises during Passover. (I'll bet her husband's happy.)

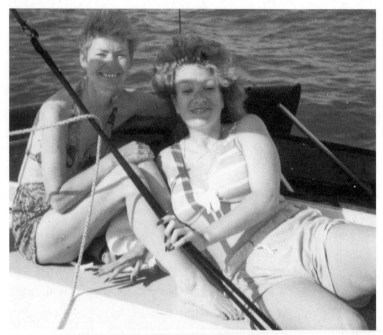

Me and Mom in Florida… The Toni Twins!

THIRTEEN

Odds and (Rear) Ends

Answering all those questions inspired me to add this final chapter, which actually is a collection of thoughts that would remain random if not for this book.

Like all fat people, I'm constantly pestered by skinny people. (Why is it that skinny people automatically assume that just because you look like you're related to Orson Welles that they can insult you by asking the dumbest questions you've ever heard?)

Just the other day, a skinny person came up to me and asked the all-time, number-one-ranked stupid question, the one that really, really pisses me off: "Why did you gain all that weight?" the Q-tip asked innocently, in that whiny, little voice that skinny people have—the one that lets you know that the only reason they asked is so that they can gloat over how much thinner than you they are.

To begin with, none of us know WHY we gained the weight. If we did, then it would be a hell of a lot easier to lose that stuff. Plus, there's never a simple explanation as to why we did it. Even when it looks like the reason is a simple one, such as a failed relationship, a death in the family, or—in my case—because they opened a Taco Bell next door to my apartment, it isn't simple. In other words, this is a stupid question from the very start, to say nothing of the fact that it's rude, annoying, and—if it comes from a spouse—grounds for divorce in most states.

So after this skinny person asked me WHY I was so fat, you can imagine how angry I was. But I dealt with the situation, and if you use the following technique, you'll be able to deal with it, too.

First, I took 10 deep breaths. Of course, that was just to get enough energy to stand up. (I was seated at the time and I wanted to be able to look this stupid skinny person in the eye while I cussed her out.) Once I was face to face with the offender, I first asked her if she was born dumb, or if she had made it a life-long project to get that way. The glazed look in her eye pretty much answered the question, so then I let her have it.

"I gained all this weight," I said, "because I am fascinated by the amazing selection of clothes in the fat-lady stores; I never want another date; I crave low self-esteem; and, most of all, if I was thin I'd miss all those spellbinding conversations with YOU!"

You won't make any friends with this technique, but trust me, it will make you feel a lot better about yourself. Plus, who wants thin friends? It's not a long-term solution, mind you, but in the short run, the ego boost it provides is roughly equivalent to wolfing down 10 Twinkies or an entire bowl of cake batter. Anger—it's the best calorie saver I know of...

...Sometimes the stupid questions don't come from skinny people—they come from old friends and relatives who haven't seen you since you put on the 80 or so pounds that are keeping you from looking like your old, human-sized self. Bear in mind, these people will be incredibly alarmed by the sight of you, and rightfully so. No one told them that you're now large enough to be mistaken for one of those mascots that roam the sidelines at professional sporting events, and they'll probably think you're wearing some kind of costume. Or maybe they'll just assume that you finally decided to fulfill your life-long dream of becoming a professional wrestler.

Trust me, it can happen. After all, most of the clothes at fat-lady stores are basically identical to the outfits you see in pro wrestling, what with all the sequins, glitter, and garish colors. In fact, after a day of shopping at Lane Giant, all you need is a nickname and a trainer, and you'll be ready for the next Wrestlemania.

So when it's been 15 years and you run into your long-lost cousin—or for that matter, your husband—don't be alarmed when they look frightened. Be prepared. First, they'll probably shriek out loud, turn ashen, and run for the hills. In fact, if you're meeting an elderly relative, you might want to have a doctor standing by. After your beloved family members take their heart medication and calm down a bit, they'll inevitably feel compelled to ask the big question. Much as manners, good taste, and just plain old human decency dictate otherwise, they won't be able to avoid blurting out, "WHAT THE HELL HAPPENED TO YOU?"

There's not really a delicate way for your loved ones to ask this question, so don't worry about answering it delicately either. Just tell them the truth: "Well, I got sick and tired of being ogled by gorgeous men and envied by all women. Perky, firm, self-supporting breasts were becoming a drag and, basically, I got tired of feeling good all the time. I mean, how many rock stars can you turn down and still respect yourself? I much prefer living life this way, where I get so winded from going outside to get the mail that I have to take a nap. Plus, it's just a kick to look pregnant all the time."

This should keep them quiet for awhile. And by the way, when it comes to relatives, avoid children AT ALL COSTS. The little weasels know how to tell the truth and believe me, that's the last thing any fat person wants to hear. Instead of lying to you and saying something like, "Gosh, no, that circus tent you're wearing looks great—the stripes really suit you," little Timmy will say, "Mommy, when did (INSERT YOUR NAME HERE) turn into such a big, fat load?"...

...One of my favorite things to do when I'm sleeping with the one I love is to "spoon," which is when you lie on your sides back-to-front and cradle each other. Once I was on the road and working in Nashville, and I spent a long and loving night being the outside spoon. There I was, lying with my love all night, feeling the warmth and comfort that he provides, and enjoying every moment of it. Until I woke up and realized I was ALONE! I'd spent the evening with my arm around MY OWN STOMACH, which was so big, I actually thought it was another person...

...The silliest date I've ever been on took place several years ago. After spending years trying to get this one guy to take me out, it finally happened. So of course I put on my TIGHTEST jeans. I was sitting at the bar with this great guy, and all of a sudden I felt my zipper just BURST open—zipper, crotch, butt—EVERY-THING! I had to sit at the bar for HOURS, because I knew if I got up I'd be dead. Of course, when you're sitting at the bar that long, you don't have any choice but to keep ordering drinks. So the longer I sat there, the drunker I got and the worse I had to go to the bathroom. I don't remember how I got out of that one, but suffice it to say that when you park it by the bar all night, it doesn't really matter if you're wearing pants or not when you get up to go home...

...I looked down the other day and realized that my ankles HAD TURNED INTO PAINT CANS!!. Would someone please tell me exactly WHEN this happened and HOW LONG I've been walking around looking like this? (The problem is, I can't actually see my ankles. I just happened to catch a glimpse of their reflection in my right rear hubcap.) I swear, I used to have slim, beautiful ankles, and now I look like I'm hauling around a couple of cans of The Weatherbeater. And it's going to take a lot more than two cans of paint to cover my surface area!...

...When you take antidepressants, aside from gaining 600 pounds—which is bound to cheer anyone up—you SWEAT like a madman going to The Chair. Even if you don't drink anything all day, your body still will produce enough water to fill one of those blow-up kiddie pools—not that you'll be able to fit into one...

...If you're fat, I don't recommend para-sailing. Floating in the sky about 100 feet above water from a parachute that's pulled behind a boat is the most exhilarating thing I've ever done, but I made the mistake of having it videotaped. The cameraperson films you going up and coming down, and the poor soul has no choice but to shoot you BUTT FIRST! When I got home and popped the videotape into the VCR, it was the scariest thing I'd ever seen in my life. Let me tell you, when it comes to shock value, para-sailing itself can't hold a candle to that video. All you could see was my big butt on TV roaring toward the camera. Talk about Faces of Death!...

...One last fashion tip: NEVER, NEVER, NEVER wear white. You'll look like Moby Nurse. Nothing in the world makes you look fatter than white—with the possible exception of full frontal nudity, but where I live they don't really go for that sort of thing, even from the hardbodies. I know you all want to go for that popular waif look, but the bad news is, if you're even 8 ounces overweight, YOU CAN'T HAVE IT! So ladies, stick with black, black, black. BUT NO SPANDEX!...

...If you don't think I know what you as a fat person are going through, then listen to this: While writing this book, I have lost and gained back 20 pounds. So trust me, I know what your life is like.

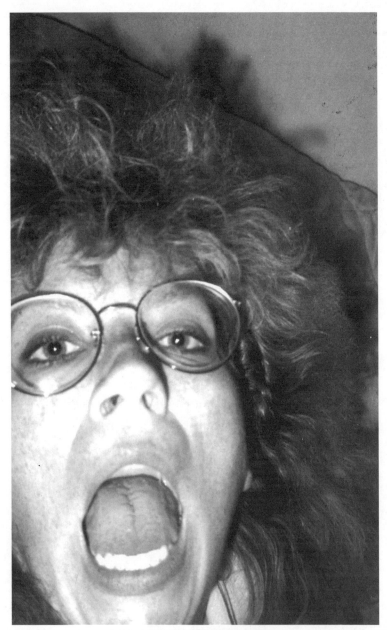

The view for a loaf of garlic bread.

Afterword

As I sit here finishing this book, I want to add one final anecdote, something that happened to me just a few weeks ago. I was called quite suddenly to Los Angeles to audition as a supporting player for a new sitcom that will appear on ABC this fall.

When I went into the audition, all the other girls were skinny and perfect. After the reading, which went very well, I asked my manager if the producer had said anything about my weight. I was really worried, especially since I knew I was up against nothing but stick figures. But my manager put me at ease. He told me they loved me, and then he explained what he meant. "Don't worry, they liked you just like you were," he said. "They don't want the audience to think that the male star could be romantically interested in you."

Great. Thanks, I think.

Turns out I didn't get the part; I just couldn't seem to convince them that chunky is "in." Gotta go, my stomach is growling…